Advances in Behavioral Pharmacology

VOLUME 7

ADVANCES IN BEHAVIORAL PHARMACOLOGY

A series of volumes edited by:
Travis Thompson, Peter B. Dews, James E. Barrett

KRASNEGOR, GRAY, THOMPSON • *Developmental Behavioral Pharmacology, Vol. 5*

THOMPSON, DEWS, BARRETT • *Neurobehavioral Pharmacology, Vol. 6*

BARRETT, THOMPSON, DEWS • *Advances in Behavioral Pharmacology, Vol. 7*

Advances in Behavioral Pharmacology

VOLUME 7

Edited by

JAMES E. BARRETT

Department of Psychiatry
Uniformed Services University of the
* Health Sciences School of Medicine*
Bethesda, Maryland

TRAVIS THOMPSON

Department of Psychology
University of Minnesota
Minneapolis, Minnesota

PETER B. DEWS

Department of Psychiatry
Harvard Medical School
Boston, Massachusetts

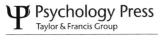 Psychology Press
Taylor & Francis Group

New York London

First Published by

Lawrence Erlbaum Associates, Inc., Publishers
10 Industrial Avenue
Mahwah, New Jersey 07430

Transferred to Digital Printing 2009 by Psychology Press
270 Madison Ave, New York NY 10016
27 Church Road, Hove, East Sussex, BN3 2FA

Library of Congress Catalog Card Number: 74-10147

ISBN 0-8058-0351-3
ISSN 0147-071X

Publisher's Note
The publisher has gone to great lengths to ensure the quality of this
reprint but points out that some imperfections in the original may be apparent.

Contents

Contributors To This Volume   viii

Preface   ix

Chapter 1   **BEHAVIORAL PHARMACOLOGY: ISSUES OF
REDUCTIONISM AND CAUSALITY**   1
M. Jackson Marr

References   11

Chapter 2   **EFFECTS OF DRUGS ON STIMULUS CONTROL
OF BEHAVIOR UNDER SCHEDULES OF
REINFORCEMENT**   13
Jonathan L. Katz

Introduction   13
Methods   17
Effects of Drugs on Response Rates and
Stimulus Control Under Fixed-Interval
Schedules   19
Comparison of Free Operant and Discrete
Trials Procedures   23
Generality of Effects of Fixed-Interval
Responding   24
Analysis of the Source of Stimulus Control
Altered by Drugs   28
Summary and Implications   32
References   37

Chapter 3 **CONTRIBUTIONS OF THE MATCHING LAW TO THE ANALYSIS OF THE BEHAVIORAL EFFECTS OF DRUGS** 39
Gene M. Heyman, Michael M. Monaghan

Introduction 39
The Problem of Measuring a Subject's Susceptibility to Reinforcers 40
The Matching Law Equation: Basic Findings 41
Neuroleptics 46
Amphetamine 58
Antidepressants 66
New Directions: Avoidance Responding 67
Caveats and Summary 70
References 73

Chapter 4 **BEHAVIORAL PHARMACOLOGY OF COMPOUNDS AFFECTING MUSCARINIC CHOLINERGIC RECEPTORS** 79
Jeffrey M. Witkin

Introduction 79
Cholinesterase Inhibitors and Muscarinic Agonists 82
Muscarinic Antagonists 95
Muscarinic Receptor Subtypes 106
Conclusions 112
References 113

Chapter 5 **BEHAVIORAL RESPONSES ASSOCIATED WITH SEROTONIN RECEPTORS** 119
Irwin Lucki

Multiple Types of 5-HT Receptors 120
Unconditioned Behaviors Elicited by 5-HT Agonists 121
Regulation of Behavioral Responses Elicited by 5-HT Agonists 131
Drug Discrimination Studies 137
5-HT Receptor Subtypes and Behavior 138
Summary 140
References 141

Chapter 6   **NUTRITIONAL ASPECTS OF DRUG ACTION ON BEHAVIOR**   **149**
Kathleen M. Kantak

Introduction   149
Tryptophan   150
Magnesium   155
Ascorbic Acid   161
Conclusions   163
References   165

Chapter 7   **ROLES AND CHARACTERISTICS OF THEORY IN BEHAVIORAL PHARMACOLOGY**   **171**
Marc N. Branch, David W. Schaal

The Domain of Behavioral Pharmacology   172
Theories: Their Roles and Characteristics   174
Behavioristic Theory   179
The Nature of a Theory for Behavioral
  Pharmacology   183
The Prospects for a Theory   192
References   193

Author Index   197
Subject Index   207

Contributors To This Volume

MARC N. BRANCH • Department of Psychology, University of Florida, Gainesville, FL 32611

GENE M. HEYMAN • Department of Psychology, Harvard University, Cambridge, MA 02138

KATHLEEN M. KANTAK • Department of Psychology, Boston University, Boston, MA 02215

JONATHAN L. KATZ • NIDA Addiction Research Center, P.O. Box 5180, Baltimore, MD 21224

IRWIN LUCKI • Department of Psychiatry, Behavioral Pharmacology Laboratory, University of Pennsylvania, Philadelphia, PA 19104

M. JACKSON MARR • School of Psychology, Georgia Institute of Technology, Atlanta, GA 30332

JEFFREY M. WITKIN • NIDA Addiction Research Center, P.O. Box 5180, Baltimore, MD 21224

Preface

Advances in Behavioral Pharmacology continues with this volume to address new issues and topics, while recognizing the continuity and clear contributions from the past. The current volume embraces issues of behavioral pharmacology important to its foundation and emergence as a scientific discipline and scientific growth (Marr, Branch and Schaal), and also provides an analysis of a topic of long-standing central import to behavioral pharmacology, that of stimulus control (Katz). The growing use of behavioral techniques to analyze effects of drugs interacting with specific neurotransmitter systems (Witkin and Lucki) is still further testimony to the importance of integrating behavior and neuropharmacological analyses. Relatively new areas of research are represented by chapters on the matching law (Hyman) and on nutritional aspects contributing to the behavioral effects of drugs (Kantak). This collection of chapters then, although heterogeneous, is an appropriate means of highlighting both recurring and emerging themes in behavioral pharmacology.

ACKNOWLEDGMENTS

We would like to express our sincere appreciation to Bristol-Myers, DuPont and Pfizer for their generous support in the production of this volume. Without their support, it would have been impossible to proceed. We hope this volume recognizes in some small way the important interplay between drug development and behavior and look forward to a special volume specifically on this issue.

T.T., Minneapolis
P.B.D., Cambridge
J.E.B., Bethesda

1 Behavioral Pharmacology: Issues of Reductionism and Causality

M. Jackson Marr

Georgia Institute of Technology

Behavioral pharmacology is now over 3 decades old. In 1955 Peter Dews published his article "Differential sensitivity to pentobarbitol of pecking performance in pigeons depending upon the schedule of reward." This epoch-making study, whose implications have yet to be fully fathomed, emerged from a contact between Peter Dews, a pharmacologist at Harvard Medical School and B. F. Skinner's laboratory across the river in Cambridge, then peopled by such talented researchers as William Morse, Charles Ferster, and Richard Herrnstein. Morse was soon to join Peter Dews' laboratory, to be joined later by Roger Kelleher, and the trio of Dews, Morse, and Kelleher and their academic offspring were to provide a headwater of principles and research methods that remain in the mainstream of behavioral pharmacological investigation. But these proximal historical details obscure the distal, but deeper influences. The two disciplines whose confluence yielded behavioral pharmacology, namely the experimental analysis of behavior and pharmacology, have a common methodological origin in the classical physiology of Claude Bernard (1957). This has been emphasized by Travis Thompson (1984) in his retrospective review of Bernard's *An Introduction to the Study of Experimental Medicine* wherein he says:

> The experimental analysis of behavior has typically had its academic home in the discipline of psychology. Paradoxically, the experimental analysis of behavior shares much more with the tradition of Claude Bernard than it does with those of Wundt or Freud. Indeed, if an 19th century progenitor of contemporary behavior-analytic theory were to be identified, it would be Bernard and not, as is often claimed, James or Pavlov. James' pragmatism and Pavlov's reflexology were

1

peripheral to the metatheoretical and theoretical foundations of modern behavior-analytic theory and practice. (p. 211)

And, as I have said elsewhere: "The animal chamber and the cumulative recorder, as ingenious as they are, are direct descendents of the dissecting table and the smoked drum" (Marr, 1984, p. 358).

Bernard may also be credited with important developments in basic pharmacological method and theory as exemplified by his famous studies of the actions of curare. His experimental demonstration that curare had a physiological *locus* of action was to have powerful implications for pharmacology in general. Methodologically, he emphasized the value of techniques we now call the "ABA design" and "systematic replication" (Bernard, 1957; Sidman, 1960).

The level of analysis of Bernard's physiology, that is, the focus on organ and tissue function is also reflective of both classical pharmacology and the modern experimental analysis of behavior. It is easy to make the correspondence between the study of organ and tissue function on the one hand and, on the other hand, the rate and pattern of keypecks and the sequence or distribution of interresponse times.

The experimental analysis of behavior has provided orderly and repeatable data on the actions of individual organisms. The data are subject to the most compelling visual display as well as detailed quantitative scrutiny. So it was with physiological investigation of organ and tissue systems. The rate and pattern of the heartbeat, the response of an isolated smooth muscle to electrical or chemical stimulation, and yes, the secretion of saliva, all represent orderly phenomena subject to the prediction and control inherent in a functional analysis. Pharmacology advanced by the study of the effects of drugs on these kinds of response systems.

Consideration of the axiom that behavior is a biological property of organisms, coupled with the orderly data that can emerge from an appropriate behavioral analysis leads one to consider the significance of the study of the effects of drugs on behavior, or, more precisely, drug-behavior interactions. This reasoning, however, is both glib and formal and requires a more careful consideration of what might be termed the *causal structure* of the field of investigation. That is, the relationships and their directions holding between variables of one class, say pharmacological, and variables of another class, say behavioral. This causal structure is reflective of the rationale and methods for investigation. It constitutes the texture of functional relations and in a sense is descriptive of the consequences maintaining the behavior of the investigator.

Causal structure also embodies the levels of analysis that can enter into an account, that is, characteristic reductive modes. The term "reduction" itself plays a number of complex roles in the language games of science, no doubt a major source of the vigorous controversies engendered by the term. Ernest Nagel (1979) provided a framework concerning the logic of reductive explanations which is useful for exploring the reductive aspects of the causal structure of drug-behavior interations.

Nagel distinguished two forms of reductionism: homogeneous and heterogeneous. A formal paradigm for *homogeneous reduction* is the deduction from a general theory of implications (or theorems) in which there is a communality of terms. For example, the cosmos of Kepler and the kinematics of Galileo are deducible from Newtonian laws. Moreover, there is a common terminology: velocity, mass, acceleration, etc., or, more generally, a common set of variables entering into functional relations. In contrast, *heterogeneous reduction* embodies what Skinner (1950) described as "any explanation of an observed fact which appeals to events taking place somewhere else, at some other level of observation, described in different terms, and measured, if at all, in different dimensions" (p. 193).

Nagel's category of homogeneous reductionism explanation is more familiar to behavior analysts. The matching law and its cousins, and various formulations of reinforcing principles are representatives. Ferster and Skinner's (1957) analysis of schedules of reinforcement is based on conditions prevailing at the moment of reinforcement; and concepts of response strength and probability of reinforcement per response have represented basic formulations of behavior from which the characteristic aspects of behavior are assessed or derived. A common set of variables and terms, e.g., reinforcement, reinforcement frequency, rate, patterns of interresponse times, prevail.

The concern with "units of behavior" or the "molar *vs.* molecular" issue would appear to entail the heterogeneous form of reductionism (cf. Thompson & Zeiler, 1986). However, in all cases the so-called units or the molecular components are treated as *behavioral* events. Behavior is reduced to behavior—a homogeneous reduction after all.

One of the most general "covering laws" of behavioral pharmacology is the notion of *rate dependency,* (or *rate constancy,* if you prefer), i.e., that the rate of responding is an important determiner of a drug effect. Again, the effects of a drug on behavior is explained by reference only to a behavioral variable—rate. A large variety of experiments and observations has been interpreted in the context of this principle. It has been questioned from several quarters, most recently by Branch (1984); but it could be argued that for better or worse, it is, or has been, the only general integrative principle in behavioral pharmacology. But perhaps things are not all that bleak. Through vigorous and careful experimental analysis, salient variables and functional relations at the behavioral level have emerged that could provide for effective prediction and interpretation of drug-behavior interactions without the necessity to engage in shifts in levels of analysis. An example is the investigation of the stimulus properties of drugs which has evoked principles of stimulus control in the interpretation and classification of drug effects on behavior.

The formative model for causal structure in the physiology-pharmacology axis has provided analogs in the behavior-pharmacology axis. The formulation of a causal structure for the physiology-pharmacology axis is constructed from the investigation of the question "What does a drug do to the activities of an organ or tissue?" For example, how does a drug affect the rate and pattern of the heartbeat? The causal structure begins to take form from additional questions derived from simply showing the drug *has* an effect: "What do the drug effects tell us about the mechanisms of action?"; "What do the drug effects tell us about the drug, i.e., how the drug might be classified?"; and, "What do the drug effects tell us about the physiology of the organ system?"

These questions do not, of course, exhaust the possibilities. The form, range, and depth of such questions depend on the theoretical and methodological framework of the related fields, their knowledge bases, and the levels of analysis to which (or from which) explanatory appeals are directed.

Comparable questions arise as to the relations between behavioral and pharmacological variables. Thus: "What does a drug do to behavior?"; "What variables control these effects?"; "What do the effects on behavior tell us about the mechanism of action of the drug?"; and, "What do the drug effects tell us about behavior?" The answers to such questions will depend minimally on what is meant by *behavior,* entailing an entire philosophical and methodological approach. The foregoing questions might have been very different or, at least very differently stated. Likewise, "mechanism of action" is in itself an ambiguous phrase to which one might respond with behavioral, physiological, biochemical or even molecular relationships.

Consider the practice of describing the behavioral effects of drugs in such heterogeneous reductive modes as alterations in emotional, motivational or perceptive states, excitatory or inhibitory processes and the like. However, the experimental analysis of behavior, as manifested in behavioral pharmacology, has eschewed these kinds of expressions and has focused upon functional relations wherein changes in behaviors (e.g., keypecks, lever presses, verbal responses) are expressed in terms of such directly manipulatable variables as (1) schedule arrangement, (2) rate of responding, (3) consequences, (4) context, (5) drug history, and (6) behavioral history. Thus, answers to the question "What does a drug do to behavior?" are, first of all, generally constrained to statements about relative probabilities of actions and their distributions in time. This is in conformity with the old pharmacological principle that drugs do not confer *new* physiological, and by extension, behavioral properties or processes; they can only modify, i.e., enhance, reduce, or alter the frequency or pattern of a given function. As Peter Dews (1964) once expressed it: "Drugs change the temporal patterns of force development by the heart; they do not make the heart secrete urine" (p. 200). This is congruent with a homogeneous reductive perspective. However, physiological or behavioral changes may possibly emerge from the presence of *new combinations of molecular structures* in which the drug participated directly or indirectly as, for example, by agents that alter genetic mechanisms.

The six variables cited earlier are said to control the effects of drugs on behavior; that is, changes in behavior are functions of control rate, schedule arrangement, etc., separately, or in interactive combination. *In this analysis, the drug can be looked upon as simply another environment or historical manipulation.* This is perhaps most clearly exemplified by the study of the stimulus properties of drugs. These investigations demonstrate that, like other environmental events, drugs may act as reinforcing, punishing, eliciting, or discriminative stimuli. Such studies have both basic and applied value for the classification of drugs and for extensions of the principles of stimulus control gained through the experimental analysis of behavior in the absence of drugs.

The behavior analyst manipulates environmental variables with the ultimate consequence of developing a systematic, functional account of behavior. Because the imposition of a drug may be treated as another class of environmental manipulations, as suggested earlier, it follows that this manipulation might prove useful for the analysis of behavior. This aspect of behavioral pharmacology has not received the attention it deserves, yet for *behavior analysts* it should provide one of the most compelling rationales for the investigation of drug-behavior interactions. Drug effects can enlighten our understanding of behavior as well as reveal our naivete. As an example of the latter, punishment is usually defined as a consequence of responding that suppresses responding (Arzin & Holz, 1966). Certain drugs diminish the suppressive effects of punishing events, an important effect in the screening of putative anxiolytic agents. Yet as Branch, Nicolson, and Dworkin (1977) have shown, suppressive effects of some events, e.g., time outs or brief stimuli associated with periods of nonreinforcement, are *not* reduced by the usual anxiolytics. Just as "all that glisters is not gold," "all that suppresses is not punishment," at least from a pharmacological perspective.

The spectre of *heterogeneous reductionism* gestates in questions of the form: "What do the *mechanism of action of drugs* tell us about their effects on behavior?"; or "What do behavioral effects of drugs tell us about the *mechanism of action of drugs?*"; and, perhaps most fundamentally: "What do the *mechanisms of action of drugs* tell us about the *mechanism of actions of behavior?*"

What one means by "mechanisms of action" will, or course, depend on whether one accepts the value of a homogeneous reductive explanation or, conversely, exclusively pursues explanatory schemes at other levels. (One might engage in the diplomatic flight to parallelism, but then the issue of relationships between drug and behavioral mechanisms of action seems to lose its meaning.) We leave the world of homogeneous explanations when we no longer view a drug as an aspect of the environment or as an "establishing operation," to use Michael's term. Beyond these roles, a drug must then be viewed as a modifier of physiological or biochemical processes. The "pharmacology" in behavioral pharmacology then asserts itself. As mentioned earlier, classical pharmacology essentially shared its methods and levels of analysis with classical physiology. Following the views of Claude Bernard, neither science could have been said to be reductionistic in the heterogeneous sense. But modern physiology and pharmacology share in the general fund of biological explanation of which there are at least five aspects: (1) biochemical/biophysical; (2) physiological (i.e., organ and tissue function); (3) morphogenic-developmental; (4) behavioral–environmental; and (5) species adaptation and evolution.

The expansion of the explanatory horizon for pharmacology had its origins in the dawn of the field. Paracelsus had asserted boldly: "The body is made of chemicals, and its ills should be treated by chemicals." But true enlightenment as regards mechanism had to wait some 300 years for Bernard (with some irony) and Erlich and Langley to propose in various ways the concept of *receptor*. The receptor is one of those rare hypothetical constructs that made good. Only the concepts of atom and gene have had greater success in the scientific venture. The hypothetical nature of the receptor has largely vanished to be replaced by the quantum mechanics of molecular structure and now all of basic pharmacology must pay tribute to it. The receptor is *the* integrative principle of pharmacology and the effect on behavioral pharmacology has been profound. Behavior has now become *tissue*—a kind of clam heart or frog rectus muscle—for the assessment of drug-receptor interaction. A review of this role in the armamentarium of the pharmacologist demonstrates first of all behavior's place as another isolatable biological feature of the organism. Second, the use of behavior as tissue provides results which are, generally, on equal standing with organ, tissue or other *in vivo* or *in vitro* methods—both in terms of ease and of difficulty of interpretation. For example, behavioral techniques have played a major role in the analysis and classification of opiate receptor activation and antagonism. The volume edited by Seiden and Balster, *Behavior Pharmacology: The Current Status* (1985) contains several papers illustrating the empirical and conceptual elegance of this work.

Woods and his colleagues (1985) have applied drug discrimination procedures to assess the effects of binding to opiate receptors of certain opiate antagonists such as buprenorphine, beta-funaltrexamine, and beta-chlornaltrexamine. The goal of this work was to compare behavioral procedures and *in vitro* methods in terms of the usual criteria for irreversible binding to receptors. The outcome is that no one method, *in vitro* or *in vivo* (e.g., behavioral) provides definitive evidence and the results of different methods may in conflict. However, consistent results are available in certain cases, yielding *convergent* evidence for irreversible binding.

Both *in vitro* and *in vivo* procedures are also required to distinguish the various categories of opiate receptors—mu, kappa, and sigma—as illustrated by the work of Holzman (1985) and Leander (1985). Each receptor is identified by a *constellation* of effects—physiological, pharmacological, and behavioral. While no one of these stands out as *the* reductive marker, a behavioral distinction would seem essential, because opiates (and many other drugs) are, after all, of interest primarily because they affect behavior.

Drugs are often classified in terms of what appear to be a dominant therapeutic or toxic effect. Such an effect may only be that which is considered useful on the one hand or dangerous on the other—stimulant, depressant, antidepressant, tranquilizer, anxiolytic, convulsant, poison, euphoriant, analgesic—represent just a small set of "generic" descriptions. To view drugs as having only a single effect is, of course, naive. The "effect" of a curare-like agent will depend on whether you are a Jivaro Indian in the Amazon headwaters foraging for food with a blowgun, or a surgeon concerned with muscular spasms during an abdominal procedure. The notion of a single "generic" effect is, in part, an outcome of heterogeneous reductive thinking—as if Erlich's concept of "the magic bullet" were to be taken all too seriously. One could then speak of *the* mechanism of action of a drug, meaning a specific physiological/biochemical action. However, even if we focus on a particular effect, assuming we can adequately characterize what is meant by that effect—not a trivial problem when it comes to clinical description, or to the development of laboratory models—we find that the drug effect of interest may be controlled or modulated by numerous *behavioral* variables. Dykstra (1985) reviewed the role of behavioral variables in the analgesic action of opiates. Stimulus intensity, type of stimulus, response rate, and schedule were found to be significant determinants of variation in analgesic effects. These same variables, along with others, would play significant roles in *all* the generic categories and implied effects noted earlier. But, one can go much further. Drugs alter the physiological/biochemical environment. As already mentioned, such alterations do not imply new functions, but rather modulation of already established functions. For example, the notion of endogenous opiate or anxiolytic receptors embodies this principle. There are other sources besides drugs for such modulations, both endogenous and exogenous. Endogenously, for example, there are numerous complex rhythms of hormones, physiological functions, and other body constituents. Exogenously, one could consider the food and other substances we take in or, more in a research or clinical context, to the numerous procedures for physiological alteration from hormone administration to brain lesions—the effects of *all* of these are subject to the categories of behavioral variables known to modulate drug effects. Behavior-environment variables and interactions thus take a significant and unique place in a community of biological explanations.

One might well ask, however, whether this community is a loose confederation or a centralized federation. The latter is founded on a "unity of science" concept, with a hierarchy of levels, each reduced to the one "below" it in the heterogeneous reductive sense. Perhaps the evolution of the human species, and my behavior involved in writing this article about reductionism, could be described, predicted, and ultimately controlled, in *principle,* by the adroit application of the laws of quantum field theory. (I do not wish to explore here the interesting implications of the view of some Idealists and others that physics is really a branch of psychology!) There are those who could argue persuasively that behavior is not only reducible to physics by various causal links, but is *identical* with certain physical states. In behavioral pharmacology, we might inquire, whether the pattern of behaviors we classify as "analgesia" is *identical* with the activation of opiate receptors. Clearly not, although opiate receptor activation may be a component of an opiate-related analgesia as opposed, say, to aspirin-related analgesia. Many other variables contribute to the effect. Perhaps the collection of those variables could ultimately be described by the activation of many different kinds of receptors. Indeed, some experimental efforts have been made to characterize particular behaviors by hormonal or neural transmitter states and relate these to differential drug effects.

Although Bernard emphasized the value of focusing upon the organ-tissue aspect of biological function, his vigorous assertions of antivitalism gave support to the thesis that all life processes were physiochemical in nature, subject to deterministic laws. Skinner was to do likewise. He attempted to drive the spirits of animism and mentalism—homunculi, ghosts in the machine, mental states, etc., out of the temple of behavior, and at the same time to emphasize that behavior is subject to deterministic functional relations between the variables of history, contingency, context, and behavior itself. Skinner has, however, maintained a complex view of heterogeneous reductionism, asserting that behavior deserved its own place in the scientific sun (what Bernard had also said about physiology). Skinner (1974) is especially contemptuous of *neurologizing*—the view that behavioral events must be stated in conceptual neural terms, hypothetical constructs and the like. As to the role of *real* physiology/biochemical science and its relation to behavioral analysis, his concerns have been more pragmatic:

> The theory of knowledge called Physicalism holds that when we introspect or have feelings we are looking at states or activities of our brains. But the major difficulties are practical: we cannot anticipate what a person will do by looking directly at his feelings or his nervous system, nor can we change his behavior by changing his mind or his brain. (p. 11)

As previously emphasized, explanation in the experimental analysis of behavior operates in a homogeneous reductive mode in that causal structure is embodied in a specification of the controlling variables of behavior which, in turn, enter into an organized set of functional relations. Functional relations can have the property that the *direction* of causality is merely a reflection of emphasis, a characteristic considered by many to be a principal weakness of a purely functional account. Thus one might focus on how differences in reinforcement frequency affect how a drug changes rate; or conversely, how differences in rate affect how a drug influences reinforcement frequency. The dynamic relationships that can operate between frequency of reinforcement and rate may be said to be modulated by the imposition of the drug. These are *steady-state* relations, specifying the reversibility exemplified in the ABA design so endeared by the behavior analyst. Historical variables embodied in drug or behavioral history may or may not be reversible. In the latter case, time is provided an arrow; or, in another idiom, the *organism is changed*—certainly a most powerful temptation for trans-level (heterogeneous) reductive speculations. While a functional analyst might describe a change in an organism as a change in the behavioral repertoire (i.e., potential behavior), Skinner (1974) himself has noted there is something missing in a purely functional account:

> The physiologist of the future will tell us all that can be known about what is happening inside the behaving organism. His account will be an important advance over a behavioral analysis, because the latter is necessarily "historical"—that is to say, it is confined to functional relations showing temporal gaps. Something is done today which affects the behavior of an organism tomorrow. No matter how clearly that fact can be established, a step is missing, and we must wait for the physiologist to supply it. He will be able to show how an organism is changed when exposed to contingencies of reinforcement and only the changed organism then behaves in a different way, possibly at a much later date. What he discovers cannot invalidate the laws of a science of behavior, but it will make the picture of human action more nearly complete. (p. 215)

This is a view of the physiological/biochemical events as mediating between the environmental contingencies and behavior—a kind of *aether* mediating action at a temporal distance. The view discussed earlier of drugs serving as environmental features fits nicely here as the behavioral effects of drugs could be mediated by the physiological/biochemical aether. This view, in itself, does not necessarily imply that all drug effects or behavioral principles in general are *reducible to* physiological/biochemical events, in the sense that the laws of biophysics, biochemistry or physiology, *by themselves* yield the principles of behavior or, in turn, drug effects on behavior.

Three matters must be resolved to achieve a heterogeneous reduction. First, in order to achieve such a reduction, laws would have to contain terms or derived relations that provided bridges to, or a commonality with, statements of behavioral principles. This, in turn, is dependent upon some *theory* of the role of the reducing processes in reference to behavior, not to some putative *inherent properties* of the constituents of the reducing system. What one is actually talking about here is the verbal behavior of scientist, and not the "revealed nature" of physiological constituents. In the most successful of reductions—classical thermodynamics to kinetic theory of gases, *statements* about temperature were reduced to *statements* about the average kinetic energy of gas molecules. There are no inherent properties of molecules that would allow the observation that temperature is identical with the average kinetic energy of the molecules. So-called "emergent properties" then depend on theoretical systems adequately developed at the relevant levels which include laws to bridge one level with another. Nothing in principle prevents this possibility. Presently, however, no significant behavioral principle is derivable strictly from physiological, not to mention biochemical laws. The value of drug effects in the analysis of behavior discussed earlier derived not from known mechanisms of actions of drugs, say, at the receptor level, but rather proceeded from already established *behavioral* effects. Drugs can modify behaviors in ways not possible with other behavioral procedures. For example, they may modify rates of responding without changing reinforcement frequency or other aspects of contingencies. Why or how this occurs in a biochemical context is not considered as part of a behavioral analysis or theory.

Second, as Skinner pointed out long ago (1938), the principles of behavior will provide the framework for a physiological analysis. It was classical thermodynamics that provided the impetus for kinetic theory and statistical mechanics. Reductive explanation has always proceeded from already known principles at one level to conceptual and empirical analysis of the sub-adjacent level. We are taught to look behind a phenomenon, or perhaps *beneath* it. However, as Mercer (1981) has emphasized in an analysis of hierarchical systems in biology, each level of the hierarchy provides the boundary conditions for interpreting the laws at the sub-adjacent level. Laws are essentially useless without boundary conditions. *But the boundary conditions are not part of the laws, nor can they ever be.* To quote from Mercer:

> Complexity . . . results from placing restraints on components to introduce organizing relationships and these are boundary conditions in the physical sense. Furthermore, in complex systems organized in a hierarchical fashion, the components on a physiochemical level may be under the control of organized elements on a higher level of the hierarchy, which in this case determine the behavior at the physiochemical level. (p. 18)

Part of the boundary conditions for biological systems find their source in evolutionary processes which are essentially indeterminate in character in that the direction of evolution is not predictable from laws in the sublevels of the biological explanatory hierarchy. An important part of the boundary conditions of interest here are represented by history, context, and contingency. One might look at a drug as an additional constraint to the functioning of the physiochemical system, just as substrates impose organization upon enzyme systems. If the drug were to be considered as part of a physiochemical system, say a drug-receptor complex, then its action would still be subject to boundary conditions specified by behavioral variables.

Finally, one could argue that a physiological reduction of behavior or behavior-drug interactions would provide *simplicity*, in a Machian sense, by encompassing a wide range of facts into a small set of principles. As Skinner said more than 50 years ago ". . . I know of no simplification of behavior that can be claimed for a neurological fact" (1938, p. 425). Fifty years have not led us to revise that statement. This is not to say it will remain true. However, a perusal of Shepard's fine text, *The Synaptic Organization of the Brain* (1979), and the now classic Cooper, Bloom, and Roth (1986), suggests that the world of neurophysiology and neurochemistry is of an order of complexity far greater than it is usually given credit. A few short years ago, less than a half-dozen neural transmitters were known, and what one knew of their chemistry was confined largely to the peripheral nervous system. Now we see the brain as synthesizing, storing and releasing perhaps thousands of transmitters, hormones, modulators, etc. Synaptic action depends not simply on the special properties of these substances, but on exact geometries of fine cellular structures. The neural interactions themselves are highly nonlinear, time-dependent and, in significant cases, irreversible. Different phyla appear to have different neural organizations to carry out similar functions. Truly remarkable behaviors are exhibited by creatures with as few as 10^5 neurons, but it takes perhaps 6 orders of magnitude more cells to be able to talk about those creatures. Those calling themselves psychopharmacologists have generally focused, with good reason, on those neurochemical systems most thoroughly studied by others—acetylcholine, the catechol, and indole amines. This may be a bit like the drunk looking for his lost house key down the street where there is the most light. Perhaps this is the only feasible strategy—but some researchers in this field often remind me of Ernst Mach's (1960) comment on Descartes: ". . . a minimum of experience always suffices him for a maximum of inference" (p. 363).

Despite the dangers and limitations of heterogeneous reductionism, it is an inevitable process of the scientific enterprise. It proceeds most effectively from a careful homogeneous reduction which, in turn, provides the appropriate interpretations and explanatory scope and goals of a heterogeneous reduction. Of course, fields like behavior analysis and neurochemistry can proceed in parallel, each concerned largely, if not exclusively with its own domain. Clearly, the more knowledge gained within these separate domains, the more can be contributed by each to the construction of analytic and synthetic bridges between them. Mutual ignorance, however is only amplified by premature and grandiose attempts at synthesis and reduction.

Behavioral pharmacology seems to be in a fortunate position, bridging as it does behavior analysis with areas of pharmacology, including such supporting disciplines as neurophysiology, neurochemistry and neuroanatomy. While this arrangement is ripe for stimulation of heterogeneous reductions, as long as most significant behavioral variables are specified at the behavioral level and not really interpretable as reduced events in a physiochemical domain, behavior analysis will continue to play an essential role in our understanding of how drugs interact with biological systems.

REFERENCES

Azrin, N. H., & Holz, W. C. (1966). Punishment. In W. Honig (Ed.), *Operant behavior: Areas of research and application*. New York: Appleton-Century-Crofts.

Bernard, C. (1957). *An introduction to the study of experimental medicine* (H. C. Greene, Trans.). New York: Dover. (Original work published 1865)

Branch, M. N. (1984). Rate dependency, behavioral mechanisms, and behavioral pharmacology. *Journal of the Experimental Analysis of Behavior, 42*, 511–522.

Branch, M. N., Nicholson, G., & Dworkin, S. I. (1977). Punishment-specific effects of pentobarbital: Dependency on the type of punisher. *Journal of the Experimental Analysis of Behavior, 28*, 285–293.

Cooper, J. R., Bloom, F. E., & Roth, R. H. (1986). *The biochemical basis of neuropharmacology* (5th Ed.). New York: Oxford University Press.

Dews, P. (1955). Studies in behavior. I. Differential sensitivity to pentobarbital of pecking performance in pigeons depending on the schedule of reward. *Journal of Pharmacology and Experimental Therapeutics, 113*, 393.

Dews, P. B. (1964). Schedules of reinforcement. In H. Steinberg, A. V. S. de Reuck, & J. Knight (Eds.), *Ciba Foundation Symposium: Coordinating committees for symposia on drug action on animal behaviour and drug action*. London: J. and A. Churchill, Ltd.

Dykstra, L. A. (1985). Behavioral and pharmacological factors in opioid analgesia. In L. S. Seiden & R. L. Balster (Eds.), *Behavioral pharmacology: The current status*. New York: Alan R. Liss.

Ferster, C., & Skinner, B. F. (1957). *Schedules of reinforcement*. New York: Appleton-Century-Crofts.

Holtzman, S. (1985). Discriminative stimulus properties of opioids that interact with mu, kappa, and PCP/sigma receptors. In L. S. Seiden & R. L. Balster (Eds.), *Behavioral pharmacology: The current status*. New York: Alan R. Liss.

Leander, D. (1985). Behavioral effects of agonist and antagonist actions at kappa opioid receptors. In L. S. Seiden & R. L. Balster (Eds.), *Behavioral pharmacology: The current status*. New York: Alan R. Liss.

Mach, E. (1960). *The science of mechanics*. Homewood, IL: Open Court Press (Originally published in 1885).

Marr, M. J. (1984). Conceptual approaches and issues. *Journal of the Experimental Analysis of Behavior, 42*, 352–362.

Mercer, E. H. (1981). *The foundations of biological theory*. New York: Wiley.

Nagel, E. (1979). *The structure of science*.Indianapolis: Hackett Publishing Co.

Seiden, L. S., & Balster, R. L. (1985). *Behavioral pharmacology: The current status*. New York: Alan R. Liss.

Shepard, G. M. (1979). *The synaptic organization of the brain* (2nd Ed.). New York: Oxford University Press.

Sidman, M. (1960). *Tactics of scientific research*. New York: Basic Books.

Skinner, B. F. (1938). *The behavior of organisms*. New York: Appleton-Century-Crofts.

Skinner, B. F. (1950). Are theories of learning necessary? *Psychological Review, 57*, 193–216.

Skinner, B. F. (1974). *About behaviorism*. New York: Knopf.

Thompson, T. (1984). The examining magistrate for nature: A retrospective review of Claude Bernard's *An Introduction to the Study of Experimental Medicine*. *Journal of the Experimental Analysis of Behavior, 41*, 211–216.

Thompson, T., & Zeiler, M. (Eds.). (1986). *Analysis and integration of behavioral units*. Hillsdale, NJ: Lawrence Erlbaum Associates.

Woods, J. H., France, C. P., Bertalmino, A. J., Gmerek, D. E., & Winger, G. (1985). Behavioral assessment of insurmountable narcotic agonists. In L. S. Seiden & R. L. Balster (Eds.), *Behavioral pharmacology: The current status*. New York: Alan R. Liss.

2 Effects of Drugs on Stimulus Control of Behavior Under Schedules of Reinforcement

Jonathan L. Katz
NIDA Addiction Research Center
and
University of Maryland School of Medicine

INTRODUCTION

The initial suggestion that the effects of drugs on behavior might be due to alterations in stimulus control of responding came from a review of behavioral pharmacology by Dews (1958). In this paper, Dews suggested that the effects of drugs could depend on four classes of factors: (1) what the animal is (species and individual); (2) what the animal is doing (the response and its rate of occurrence); (3) what the environment is doing to the organism (i.e., the eliciting, reinforcing, or discriminative stimuli affecting it); and (4) what has happened to the animal in the past. Dews suggested further that many of the actions of chlorpromazine are determined by environmental (class 3) factors. More specifically, it was suggested that chlorpromazine may alter behavior by decreasing the discriminative control of behavior.

Evidence for this conclusion was provided by a study of pigeons trained to respond under a multiple fixed-interval fixed-ratio schedule. Under this schedule, responses were reinforced according to a fixed-interval schedule in the presence of blue lights and according to a fixed-ratio schedule in the presence of red lights. Once performances were stable under the schedule, distinctive performances were maintained in the presence of each stimulus (Fig. 2.1, CONTROL), indicating that the stimuli were functioning in a discriminative manner. A single dose of chlorpromazine increased rates of responding dramatically in the early portions of the fixed-interval component with little or no effects on responding during the fixed-ratio component (Fig. 2.1, 3 mg CHLORPROMA-

13

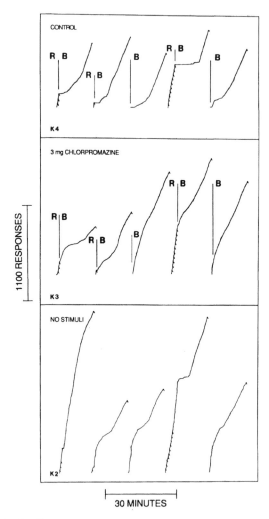

FIG. 2.1. Studies on multiple schedule performance. Each row shows
the record of a single complete day's session of the same bird. The
record on each row is continuous and has been arranged as shown
only for convenience. In the *upper* and *middle rows* the letters R and B
indicate the times when red and blue lights respectively were behind
the key. When the red light was on, each 50th response was reinforced
(shown by small diagonal hatch mark); when the blue light was on the
first response after 15 min was reinforced. In the *bottom row* for the
first time, both red and blue lights were on throughout the session,
although the sequence of reinforcement contingencies was as in previous days. Adapted from P. B. Dews (1958). Analysis of effects of
psychopharmacological agents in behavioral terms. *Federation Proceedings, 17,* 1024–1030.

ZINE). In other experiments, the individual stimuli (red or blue lights) that illuminated the response keys and functioned as discriminative stimuli during the components of the multiple schedule were illuminated during both components of the schedule. The cumulative records depicting the effects of presenting both stimulus lights (Fig. 2.1, NO STIMULI), show that this stimulus change had an effect similar to the effect of chlorpromazine, rates of responding during the early portion of the interval, which generally were low prior to drug administration were increased. Further, those rates decreased as the interval progressed and subsequently increased again (compare records labeled 3 mg CHLORPROMAZINE and NO STIMULI). The similarity of the drug effect and of rendering the discriminative stimuli indistinguishable suggested that chlorpromazine may have functioned in a manner similar to the change in discriminative stimuli, and was the primary evidence supporting the conclusion that the effects of chlorpromazine were due to a change in stimulus control. Thus, a formal similarity of the effects of the drug and the analogous environmental change was used as evidence of functional equivalence of the two effects (Dews, 1956, 1970).

Since that initial study, a number of other papers followed suggesting a role of stimulus control in the effects of chlorpromazine as well as other drugs. Dews and Morse (1961) reviewed the effects of chlorpromazine on conditioned avoidance responding. Studies showing a selective effect of chlorpromazine on avoidance responding were interpreted as an effect of the drug on the relatively weaker discriminative control of the avoidance response compared to the stronger control of the escape response. Their interpretation contrasted with the prevailing notion that chlorpromazine selectively attenuated the purported fear or anxiety motivation underlying the avoidance response and did not affect the pain motivation underlying the escape response.

Laties and Weiss (1966) compared the effects of drugs on performances maintained under fixed-interval schedules and fixed-interval schedules with stimuli associated with the passage of time (clock stimuli). With several drugs, the performances maintained under the fixed interval with the clock stimuli were disrupted less than the performances maintained under the fixed interval without the clock stimuli. These results suggested that the performances under the weaker stimulus control were affected by the drugs to a greater extent than the performances under stronger stimulus control. Similar conclusions were reached in several other papers (e.g., Laties, 1972; Rees, Wood, & Laties, 1985). These studies differed from the earlier study by Dews (1958) in that the effect of the drug was demonstrated to depend on the stimulus conditions. In contrast, Dews suggested that the effect of the drug was similar to a change in stimulus conditions.

While demonstrations that the effects of drugs can depend on stimulus conditions have been relatively straightforward, determining that the effects of drugs are similar to a change in stimulus conditions has been more difficult. One primary reason for this difficulty is that, while there are clear predictions of the form of changes in behavior expected when a drug alters stimulus control of behavior, other effects of drugs frequently predict the same formal changes in behavior. For example, stimulus control is often established by arranging different schedules of reinforcement in the presence of two stimuli. The differences in rates and patterns of responding generated by the schedules is a qualitative indication that the stimuli are controlling behavior. A change in the stimulus control of behavior would render the performances more similar. However, the effects of drugs on schedule-controlled responding are frequently characterized as rate dependent since drugs increase low response rates and decrease high response rates across a wide range of conditions (cf. Dews & Wenger, 1977). Thus, performances in the presence of two stimuli and differentiated on the basis of response rates, may be rendered more similar due to a decrease in the stimulus control of responding or due to a rate-dependent effect. Therefore, a drug effect on stimulus control of behavior and a rate-dependent effect can be indistinguishable.

The present chapter reviews a series of studies evolved from an attempt to apply measures borrowed from psychophysics (Green & Swets, 1957) to the assessment of the effects of drugs on stimulus control under schedules of reinforcement. These experiments attempted to modify the methods typically used in the study of schedule-controlled behavior only to the extent that the psychophysical measures could be applied, allowing a direct measure of the degree of stimulus control. Thus, a direct comparison could be made of the doses of drugs that affect stimulus control along with the doses that alter rates of schedule-controlled behavior, and possibly provide information relevant to a better understanding of whether the effects of drugs on schedule-controlled behavior are due to changes in stimulus control. Other studies of the effects of drugs on stimulus control of behavior have generally used discrete trials procedures and assessed whether drugs can have effects on stimulus control (see reviews by Appel & Dykstra, 1977; Heise & Milar, 1984), but not whether the effects of drugs on schedule-controlled responding are due to those effects. As is shown below, the effects of the drugs on schedule-controlled behavior in free-operant and discrete-trials procedures can be different.

Several excellent and comprehensive reviews of the literature on drug effects on stimulus control of behavior have been published (Dykstra & Genovese, 1987; Heise & Milar, 1984; Laties, 1975; Thompson, 1978). The present review differs from those as it is addressed at whether the effects of drugs on schedule-controlled behavior, as most commonly studied, can be interpreted as effects on stimulus control of behavior. Thus, the scope of this review is much more limited.

METHODS

In all the studies being reviewed, the subjects were food-deprived, White Carneau pigeons maintained at 80% of their unrestricted-feeding weights. The subjects were housed individually in home cages in which water and grit were continuously available when experimental sessions were not being conducted.

The experimental apparatus has been described in detail elsewhere (Katz, 1982). Its relevant features are as follows: Two response keys were mounted on the front wall 25.5 cm above the wire-mesh floor and each 3.0 cm from the vertical midline of the wall. Either key could be transilluminated by amber- or red-colored bulbs which were enclosed from behind so as not to emit stray light. A minimum force of 15 g on either key produced a click of a relay mounted behind the front wall and was counted as a response. A single clear bulb was centered at the top of the front wall and could provide overall chamber illumination (houselight). Food was provided by a solenoid-operated tray that could be made accessible to the subject through an opening centered on the front wall 8 cm above the floor. The chamber was enclosed within a ventilated outer shell which contained white noise to mask extraneous sounds.

During experimental sessions, the two keys were transilluminated with the different colors and the houselight was either on or off. When the houselight was on, responses on the red key were reinforced with food presentation (responses on the red key were designated S^D responses, and responses on the amber key were designated S^Δ responses). When the houselight was off, responses on the amber key were reinforced (responses on the amber key were designated S^D responses, and responses on the red key were designated S^Δ responses). Therefore, the color key on which responses were reinforced was conditional on the status (on or off) of the houselight. During different experiments, the intensity of the houselight, the number of S^Δ responses, the conditions for alternation of the keylight colors, and the conditions for alternation of the status of the houselight were varied as described below.

A schematic description of the first experiment is shown in Fig. 2.2. Responses on the S^D response key produced food according to a fixed-interval 5-min schedule. Under the fixed-interval schedule, the first S^D response after the lapse of a 5-min interval produced food. Following each food presentation, neither the houselight nor the keylights were illuminated for 60 sec (timeout). The schedule recycled after each timeout period.

All responses before the lapse of the interval, whether S^D or S^Δ, produced a 300-msec blackout of the keylights, after which the red and amber keylights were again on, however, each response randomly alternated the position of the colors of the keys. For example, after the blackout following a response with the right key illuminated red and the left key illuminated amber, the keys could be right-

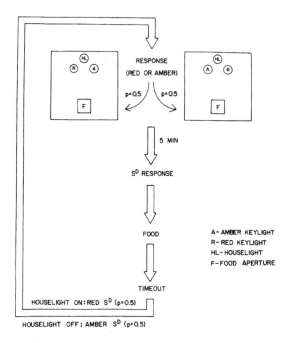

FIG. 2.2. Diagrammatic representation of fixed-interval reinforcement of responding under conditional discriminative control. Key-peck responses of pigeons on one of two keys were intermittently reinforced under a multiple fixed-interval schedule. In one component of the schedule, a houselight (HL), providing illumination of the experimental chamber, was on and responses on a red key (R) produced food according to a 5-min fixed-interval schedule. In the alternate component, the houselight was off and responses on an amber key (A) produced food, also according to a 5-min fixed-interval schedule. Each response randomly alternated the positions of the key colors (right or left) and the two components (houselight on or off) alternated in a mixed sequence. A 60 sec timeout period followed each food presentation.

red and left-amber, or right-amber and left-red, with a probability of 0.5 for either combination. The houselight was either on or off for an entire 5-min fixed-interval component. The status of the houselight (on or off) alternated in a random sequence ($p = 0.5$) with each timeout.

Stimulus control was assessed by a nonparametric statistic used for measuring sensitivity in signal detection analyses (Pollack & Norman, 1964). The statistic as applied here relates the tendency to respond appropriately in the presence of the stimulus (as represented by the proportion of S^D responses in the presence of the houselight) to the tendency to respond inappropriately in the absence of the stimulus (as represented by the proportion of S^Δ responses in the absence of the houselight). Stimulus control (A') was computed according to the formula provided by Grier (1971). In the present application, when the statistic A' is equal to 0.5, there is no stimulus control of responding (the proportion of S^D responses in the presence of the stimulus is equal to the proportion of S^Δ responses in the absence of the stimulus). When the statistic is equal to 1.0, there is perfect stimulus control (only S^D responses are emitted).

Bias for a response to one of the key colors (B''_c) as well as bias for one of the key positions (B''_p) were computed according to formulas provided by Grier (1971) and Katz (1989), respectively. Either index of bias can vary from 1.0 to -1.0, representing extreme bias towards amber or left to extreme bias towards red or right for B''_c or B''_p, respectively. A value of zero for either statistic represents no bias.

EFFECTS OF DRUGS ON RESPONSE RATES AND STIMULUS CONTROL UNDER FIXED-INTERVAL SCHEDULES

Cumulative records of performance under the multiple fixed-interval, fixed-interval schedule are shown in Fig. 2.3 (CONTROL). Responses on the red and amber keys, regardless of whether those keys were on the right or left, are represented by the top and bottom cumulative curves, respectively. The lower line was displaced downward when the houselight was off and amber was the S^D, and up when the houselight was on and red was the S^D. Rates of S^D responding were characterized by a pause followed by an increasing rate of responding up to food presentation, regardless of which key color was S^D. Rates of S^Δ responding were also characterized by a pause in the early portions of the fixed-interval followed by increases in rates. However, the rates were much lower and often decreased again as the interval progressed. The patterns of S^D responding under the fixed-interval schedule were similar to those obtained under less complex procedures in which reinforcement for a single response is scheduled according to a fixed-interval schedule (cf. Ferster & Skinner, 1957), as well as more complex procedures involving fixed-interval reinforcement of responding under conditional stimulus control (cf. Ferster, 1960).

Stimulus control, as measured by A', was generally high under control conditions; average values were 0.96 to 0.98. In addition, to determine the independence of stimulus control and response rates, both stimulus control and rates of responding were assessed in individual portions of the fixed-interval. During those portions, response rate varied over a range approximating 100 fold; across that range of response rates A' did not vary appreciably (Fig. 2.4).

The independence of stimulus control and response rates under this procedure is not entirely consistent with that reported in the literature. For example, Ferster

FIG. 2.3. Representative performances of subject N-1870 under the multiple fixed-interval schedule in which each response randomly alternated the position of the keylight colors and the status of the houselight randomly alternated during the timeout which followed each fixed-interval component. The two upper tracings within each panel show responding on the red (top) and amber (middle) response keys. The lower tracing shows the status of the houselight. When the lower event line was up, the houselight was on and responses on the red key were reinforced according to a 5-min fixed-interval schedule. When the lower event line was down, the houselight was off and responses on the amber key were reinforced according to the 5-min fixed-interval schedule. *Ordinates:* cumulative responses; *abscissas:* time. Deflections on the cumulative response records indicate presentations of food followed by the timeout during which recording stopped. Reprinted with permission from J. L. Katz (1982). Effects of drugs on stimulus control of behavior. I. Independent assessment of effects on response rates and stimulus control. *Journal of Pharmacology and Experimental Therapeutics,* 223, 617–623. © by American Society for Pharmacology and Experimental Therapeutics, 1982.

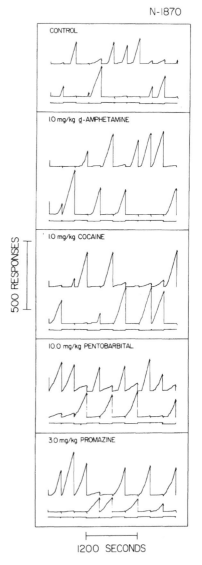

(1960) and Boren and Gollub (1972) reported some decreases in the proportion of correct responses under a conditional discrimination procedure during the middle portions of the fixed interval. These changes in accuracy may be due to differences in the procedures used or may be due, in part, to changes in bias (that contribute to the measure of accuracy used in the previous studies) rather than to changes in stimulus control.

The effects of several drugs on response rates under this conditional discrimination procedure are shown in Fig. 2.5. The psychomotor stimulants, d-amphetamine and cocaine, increased rates of S^D responding at intermediate doses, and decreased those rates at higher doses. Neither drug had appreciable effects on rates of S^Δ responding. Pentobarbital produced small increases in rates of S^D responding and also increased rates of S^Δ responding, whereas promazine produced effects that depended on the color of the response key; at some doses promazine increased rates of responding on the red key, whether S^D or S^Δ. The selected cumulative records of performance in figure 3 show that each of the drugs altered patterns of S^D responding in a manner similar to that obtained previously under fixed-interval schedules (e.g. Dews, 1958; Laties & Weiss, 1966; Rutledge & Kelleher, 1965; Smith, 1964); the low rates of responding early in the interval were increased, whereas higher rates of responding later in the interval were increased less or decreased. Thus, the effects of these drugs on the more complexly determined behavior in the present study were similar to those obtained under more conventional procedures.

Each of the drugs had little or no effects on stimulus control, as measured by A', from the lowest to relatively high doses (Fig. 2.5; filled squares). Stimulus control was decreased at the highest doses studied. Comparing the effects of these drugs on response rates and stimulus control showed that response rates

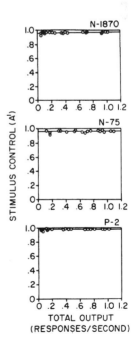

FIG. 2.4. Relations between response rates and stimulus control of responding for individual subjects studied under the fixed-interval schedule. *Abscissas:* total output of responding (rates of S^D and S^Δ responses in responses per second). *Ordinates:* Stimulus control as indicated by A'. Each point is the average value for that subject within each one min portion of each component of the multiple fixed-interval schedule. Adapted from J. L. Katz (1982). Effects of drugs on stimulus control of behavior. I. Independent assessment of effects on response rates and stimulus control. *Journal of Pharmacology and Experimental Therapeutics, 223,* 617–623.

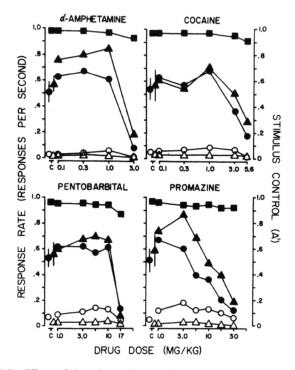

FIG. 2.5. Effects of d-amphetamine, cocaine, pentobarbital and promazine on rates of responding and A' under the multiple fixed-interval
schedule in which each response randomly alternated the position of
the keylight colors and the status of the houselight randomly alternated during the timeout which followed each fixed-interval component. *Abscissas:* drug dose (in mg/kg, log scale); *ordinates:* response
rates (responses per second) or stimulus control (A'). For explanation
of the derivation of A' see text. *Filled triangles:* S^D response rates on
the red key with houselight on; *Filled circles:* S^D response rates on the
amber key with houselight off; *Open triangles:* S^Δ response rates on
the amber key with houselight on; *Open circles:* S^Δ response rates on
the red key with houselight off; *Filled squares:* A'. Each point is the
mean of at least two observations in three subjects except control
points (above C) which are means of from 4 to 10 vehicle observations.
Vertical bars about control points represent the mean of ±1 S.D. for
each subject. Where no bars are present the point encompasses ±1
S.D. Note that the drugs only decreased A' at the highest doses that
also produced large decrements in response rates. Reprinted with permission from J. L. Katz (1982). Effects of drugs on stimulus control of
behavior. I. Independent assessment of effects on response rates and
stimulus control. *Journal of Pharmacology and Experimental Therapeutics,* 223, 617–623. © by American Society for Pharmacology and
Experimental Therapeutics, 1982.

were altered across the range of doses that had minimal effects on A'. Further, stimulus control was generally only affected at the highest doses of the drugs that produced large decreases in rates of responding.

The results of the above study suggest that the conditional discrimination procedure was closely analogous to more conventional procedures using schedule-controlled responding, since the patterns of responding maintained, and the effects of the drugs on rates of responding were similar to those typically obtained under fixed-interval schedules. Under these conditions, stimulus control remained unaffected over a range of low to intermediate doses that had effects on response rates, and was generally only decreased at the highest doses of the drugs. These doses were typically those that substantially decreased response rates. Therefore, the changes in response rate were not secondary to changes in stimulus control of responding, and a disruption in stimulus control of responding is not likely the mechanism by which these drugs alter response rates.

COMPARISON OF FREE OPERANT AND DISCRETE TRIALS PROCEDURES

In contrast to the above results, several previous studies have indicated that certain drugs can decrease stimulus control under conditional-discrimination procedures. Those studies, however, were conducted in discrete trials, matching-to-sample procedures (e.g., Berryman, Cumming, Nevin, & Jarvik, 1964) which differ from the present procedures in several respects. Thus, a subsequent study examined whether the effects obtained would depend on the type of procedure used. Subjects were studied under a discrete trials procedure similar to that diagrammed in Fig. 2.2, however, each S^D response was reinforced (fixed ratio 1-response rather than fixed-interval schedule). Each of the drugs produced dose-related decreases in rates of responding. Additionally, the effects of d-amphetamine, cocaine, and promazine on stimulus control of responding were similar to those obtained under the fixed-interval schedule (Katz, 1982). In contrast, the effects of pentobarbital on stimulus control of responding depended on the procedure used. Figure 2.6 shows that whereas pentobarbital decreased A' under the fixed-interval schedule only at the highest dose, under the fixed-ratio discrete-trials procedure stimulus control was decreased at lower doses and to a greater extent.

These results indicate that the effects of pentobarbital on stimulus control of responding depend on the conditions under which it is studied. Further, an indication that a drug alters stimulus control of behavior under one condition does not imply that the effects are generalizable to other conditions. Although discrete trials procedures indicate that an effect on stimulus control can occur, they do not indicate that the effects occur generally, or that the effect on stimulus control of behavior is a mechanism that underlies effects observed under other conditions.

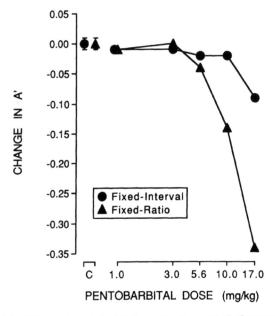

FIG. 2.6. Effects of pentobarbital on stimulus control of responding (A′) under the multiple fixed-interval schedule and under the discrete trials (fixed-ratio 1 response) procedure. *Abscissas:* drug dose (in mg/kg, log scale); *Ordinates:* stimulus control (A′). Each point is the mean of at least two observations in three (fixed-interval schedule) or two (discrete trials procedure) subjects. Vertical bars about control points represent the mean of ±1 S.D. for each subject. Note that pentobarbital only decreased A′ at the highest dose under the fixed-interval schedule, whereas pentobarbital decreased A′ at relatively lower doses under the discrete trials procedure. Adapted from J. L. Katz (1982). Effects of drugs on stimulus control of behavior. I. Independent assessment of effects on response rates and stimulus control. *Journal of Pharmacology and Experimental Therapeutics, 223,* 617–623, 1982.

GENERALITY OF EFFECTS ON FIXED-INTERVAL RESPONDING

Since the effects of pentobarbital depended on the procedure used, there may be some limits to the generality of the effects under the fixed-interval schedule. As Dews (1971) has suggested, effects of drugs on stimulus control of responding should depend on the degree of stimulus control. Thus, studies were undertaken under fixed-interval schedules to determine if the degree of stimulus control would influence the effects of the drugs.

In these studies (Katz, 1983), the procedure was identical to that diagrammed in Fig. 2.2, however the houselight intensity was systematically decreased. Decreases in the intensity of the houselight produced concomitant decreases in the value of A', and also increased the number of S^Δ responses. In most other respects control performances under this condition were similar to those described above for the fixed-interval schedule at the higher intensity houselight. The effects of d-amphetamine, cocaine, pentobarbital and promazine were again studied under fixed-interval schedules as before; however, these studies were conducted at an intensity of the houselight that produced values of A' below those obtained at the higher intensity houselight (these values averaged between 0.75 and 0.92 and showed a slow drift towards higher values the study progressed).

One major difference between the performances under the high and lower intensity houselight was the rate of S^Δ responding. Once effects of drugs were assessed at the lower intensity houselight, another study reassessed the effects of the drugs under a modified conditional-discrimination procedure which generated a higher level of S^Δ responding. This condition was similar to the fixed-interval schedule, however, a fixed number of S^Δ responses was required before an S^D response was reinforced (conjunctive schedule, Fig. 2.7). Studies of the effects of drugs under the conjunctive schedule were conducted at the higher of the houselight intensities. Under the conjunctive schedule, performances were formally equivalent to those obtained under the fixed-interval schedule at the lower intensity houselight in that rates of S^Δ responding were increased above those obtained under the fixed-interval schedule.

A comparison of the effects of the four drugs on stimulus control under the condition with the lower intensity houselight, the conjunctive schedule, and under the original conditional discrimination is shown in Fig. 2.8. The effects of both d-amphetamine and cocaine were comparable under all of the conditions studied; except at the highest doses, there were little or no effects on stimulus control. The highest doses decreased stimulus control of responding. In contrast to the effects of the psychomotor stimulants, the effects of both pentobarbital and promazine on stimulus control were greater under the fixed-interval schedule at the low intensity stimulus compared to the effects at the higher intensity stimulus (Fig. 2.8; compare squares and triangles). Further, the decreases in stimulus control were obtained at doses below those that virtually eliminated responding. Under the conjunctive schedule, the nominal values of A' were comparable to those obtained at the lower houselight intensity (Fig. 2.8; compare circles and triangles above C). However, neither drug altered A' to the degree that it was decreased under the fixed-interval schedule at the lower intensity stimulus. For example, pentobarbital produced dose-related decreases in A' at doses from 3.0 mg/kg to 17.0 mg/kg under the fixed-interval schedule at the lower intensity houselight (Fig. 2.8, triangles). In contrast, under the conjunctive schedule, the decreases in A' were much smaller in magnitude, and only occurred at doses of 10.0 and 17.0 mg/kg (Fig. 2.8, circles).

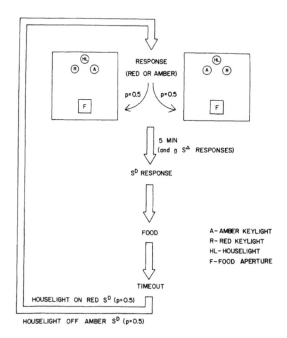

FIG. 2.7.   Diagrammatic representation of the conjunctive schedule of reinforcement. Key-peck responses of pigeons on one of two keys were intermittently reinforced under a multiple fixed-interval schedule if a minimum number of responses had been emitted on the alternate key. In one component of the schedule, a houselight (HL), providing illumination of the experimental chamber, was on and responses on a red key (R) produced food according to a 5-min fixed-interval schedule. In the alternate component, the houselight was off and responses on an amber key (A) produced food, also according to a 5-min fixed-interval schedule. Each response randomly alternated the positions of the key colors (right or left) and the two components (houselight on or off) alternated in a mixed sequence. A 60-sec timeout period followed each food presentation.

Thus, the effects of pentobarbital and promazine on stimulus control were inversely related to the degree of stimulus control over responding. Additionally, the effects were specific to weakened discriminative control produced by stimulus variables rather than merely to increased rates of S^Δ responding.

Summarizing the results of the studies reviewed to this point, under conditions in which there was a high degree of stimulus control over responding, at low to intermediate doses none of the drugs studied had appreciable effects on stimulus control of behavior. However, when the degree of control of behavior was lower, both pentobarbital and promazine decreased stimulus control of behavior. The decreases occurred at doses lower than, or comparable to those that altered rates of schedule-controlled behavior, and were not exclusively due to the changes in rates of S^{Δ} responding that accompanied the decreases in stimulus control.

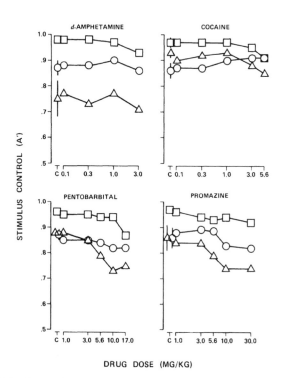

DRUG DOSE (MG/KG)

FIG. 2.8. Comparison of the effects of d-amphetamine, cocaine, pentobarbital and promazine on stimulus control of responding (A') under the multiple fixed-interval schedule at the high intensity houselight (Squares), the multiple fixed-interval schedule at the low intensity houselight (Triangles), and under the conjunctive schedule at the high intensity houselight (Circles). Abscissas: drug dose (in mg/kg, log scale); ordinates: stimulus control (A'). Note that both pentobarbital and promazine selectively decreased A' at the low-intensity houselight but did not affect comparable values of A' at a high intensity houselight under the conjunctive schedule. Reprinted with permission from J. L. Katz (1983). Effects of drugs on stimulus control of behavior. II. Degree of stimulus control as a determinant of effect. Journal of Pharmacology and Experimental Therapeutics, 226, 756–763. © by American Society for Pharmacology and Experimental Therapeutics, 1983.

ANALYSIS OF THE SOURCE OF STIMULUS CONTROL
ALTERED BY DRUGS

Subsequent studies (Katz, 1988) have analyzed further the decreases in stimulus control that can occur with d-amphetamine and pentobarbital. Under the conditional-discrimination procedure used in the studies described earlier, there were two stimuli controlling behavior: (1) the presence or absence of the houselight, and (2) the colors of the keylights. The decreases in stimulus control may have been due exclusively to changes in control exerted by the keylight colors or the houselight. Alternatively, decreases in control may have been due to changes in control exerted by both types of stimuli.

In order to determine whether the decreases in stimulus control were due to selective decreases in control by one of these types of stimuli, the effects of d-amphetamine and pentobarbital were replicated under the conditional discrimination procedure, as described in Fig. 2.2. A houselight intensity was chosen at which decreases in stimulus control of responding would be expected on the basis of the earlier findings. In the presence of the houselight, responses on the red key, regardless of position, were reinforced; in the absence of the houselight, responses on the amber key, regardless of position, were reinforced. As before, S^D responses were reinforced according to a fixed-interval 5-min schedule. Once the effects of the drugs were determined, the houselight-on and houselight-off conditions were each studied in isolation. Subjects were retrained under the houselight-on component only until the performances were stable from day to day and the effects of the two drugs were reassessed. Subsequently, the subjects were retrained under the houselight-off component and the effects of the drugs were assessed again. Under each of these subsequent conditions, the keylight colors retained their discriminative functions, since reinforcement depended on the color of the key on which the response was emitted. The houselight, however, no longer functioned as a conditional discriminative stimulus, since the key on which responses produced food did not depend on its status (on or off). In order to apply the A' statistic to these conditions, the data from these two conditions was analyzed as if they were collected simultaneously, as in the multiple schedule.

If the drugs primarily affected the control exerted by the houselight, then an effect of the drug on stimulus control would not be expected when the houselight did not function as a discriminative stimulus. Further, if the drugs primarily altered the control exerted by the keylight colors, then the effects should still have been obtained under these conditions since keylight colors still functioned as discriminative stimuli.

A comparison of the effects of pentobarbital and d-amphetamine on stimulus control under these conditions is shown in Fig. 2.9. As in the previous study (Figs. 2.5 and 2.8), d-amphetamine decreased stimulus control only at high doses which also substantially decreased response rates (Fig. 2.9; filled squares;

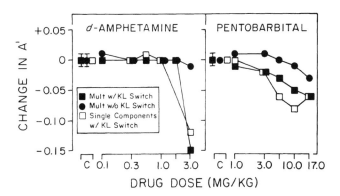

FIG. 2.9. Comparison of effects of d-amphetamine and pentobarbital on stimulus control under several different experimental conditions. *Abscissas:* drug dose (in mg/kg, log scale); *ordinates:* stimulus control (A'). *Filled squares:* multiple fixed-interval schedule in which each response randomly alternated the position of the keylight colors and the status of the houselight randomly alternated during the timeout which followed each fixed-interval component. *Open squares:* single-component fixed-interval schedules (houselight-on and -off conditions studied in isolation) in which each response randomly alternated the position of the keylight colors. *Filled circles:* multiple fixed-interval schedule in which the position of the keylight colors and the status of the houselight randomly alternated during the timeout which followed each fixed-interval component. Note that the effects off each drug were similar under the multiple schedule (filled squares) and single components (open squares), and further, the effects on stimulus control were attenuated when the positions of the keylight colors did not alternate with each response (filled circles). Adapted from J. L. Katz (1988). Effects of drugs on stimulus control of behavior. III. Analysis of the effects of d-amphetamine and pentobarbital. *Journal of Pharmacology and Experimental Therapeutics, 246:* 76–83.

left panel). In contrast, pentobarbital produced dose-related decreases in stimulus control under the multiple schedule (Fig. 2.9; filled squares; right panel). When the two components of the schedule were studied in isolation, the effects on stimulus control were similar to those obtained under the multiple schedule (Fig. 2.9; compare open and filled squares). Thus the similarity of the effects on stimulus control under the multiple schedule and the single component schedules suggests that the effects on stimulus control were due to some feature common to all three conditions. The discriminative control by the keylight colors is one such feature.

In order to further substantiate that the drugs decreased control by the keylight colors, a subsequent study was conducted in which the colors of the response keys did not randomly alternate with each response. In contrast to the previous studies in which color of the key was a unique discriminative stimulus, position of the response key could also serve as a discriminative stimulus. Thus, if discriminative control of responding by the key colors was affected, the control exerted by the position of the key might not be affected. All other aspects of the schedule were as before (Fig. 2.2); each response prior to the lapse of the fixed interval produced a 300-msec blackout of both response keys, however, the positions of the keylight colors were the same when re-illuminated; the left key was illuminated with amber and the right with red light. As in the first experiment, the houselight was either on or off for an entire 5-min fixed-interval component. The status of the houselight (on or off) alternated in a random sequence with each timeout.

Stable performances under this schedule were similar to those described previously; however, the values of A′ were, as might be expected with the additional stimulus, higher than under conditions in which the positions of the key colors alternated with each response.

At low to intermediate doses, d-amphetamine (0.1–1.0 mg/kg) produced dose-related increases in rates of S^D responding, regardless of whether the houselight was on or off. At the highest dose studied (3.0 mg/kg), response rates were decreased (Fig. 2.10, lower left panel, filled symbols). Across the range of doses studied there were no appreciable effects on rates of S^Δ responding (Fig. 2.10, lower left panel, open symbols). Across all doses studied, d-amphetamine had no effects on A′ (Fig. 2.10, upper left panel).

Pentobarbital increased rates of S^D responding in the absence of the houselight (Fig. 2.10, lower right panel, filled triangles) at 3.0 mg/kg; otherwise pentobarbital was without effects on S^D response rates with the houselight either on or off, at doses from 1.0 to 5.6 mg/kg. At the highest dose (17.0 mg/kg), S^D responding was virtually eliminated (Fig. 2.10, right panel, filled symbols). Rates of S^Δ responding in the presence or absence of the houselight were not appreciably affected across the range of pentobarbital doses studied (Fig. 2.10, lower right panel, open symbols). Doses of pentobarbital from 1.0 to 5.6 mg/kg had no effect, whereas 10.0 and 17.0 mg/kg decreased A′ (Fig. 2.10, upper right panel).

Figure 2.9 shows the effects of d-amphetamine and pentobarbital on stimulus control under this latter procedure compared to the effects under the multiple and single component schedules. As can be seen, the addition of position as a discriminative stimulus attenuated the effects of pentobarbital (right panel). With the alternation of the positions of the keylights (open and filled squares), decreases in stimulus control were greater, and obtained at doses as low as 5.6 mg/kg. With position of the keylights functioning as a discriminative stimulus (filled circles), decreases in stimulus control were attenuated, and only occurred at doses of 10.0 and 17.0 mg/kg. Decreases in stimulus control produced by d-amphetamine only occurred at high doses under the multiple and single component schedules with the keylight alternation (left panel, open and filled squares).

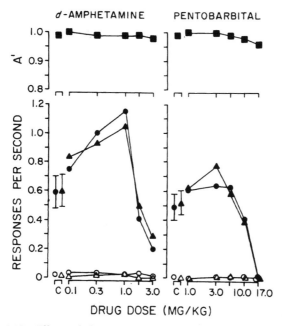

FIG. 2.10. Effects of *d*-amphetamine and pentobarbital on rates of responding and A' under the multiple fixed-interval schedule in which the position of the keylight colors and the status of the houselight randomly alternated during the timeout which followed each fixed-interval component. *Abscissas:* drug dose (in mg/kg, log scale); *ordinates:* response rates (responses per second) or stimulus control (A'). For explanation of the derivation of A' see text. Symbols are as in Fig. 2.2. Each point is the mean of at least two observations in three subjects except control points (above C) which are means of from 5 to 9 vehicle observations. Vertical bars about control points represent the mean of ±1 S.D. for each subject. Where no bars are present the point encompasses ±1 S.D. Note that *d*-amphetamine did not affect A' at any doses, whereas pentobarbital decreased A' at the highest doses. Reprinted with permission from J. L. Katz (1988). Effects of drugs on stimulus control of behavior. III. Analysis of the effects of *d*-amphetamine and pentobarbital. *Journal of Pharmacology and Experimental Therapeutics, 246,* 76–83. © by American Society for Pharmacology and Experimental Therapeutics, 1988.

These decreases were also attenuated by the addition of position as a discriminative stimulus (filled circles).

Thus, when position of the key was added to color as a discriminative stimulus, the effects of both drugs on stimulus control of behavior were attenuated. These results are consistent with the conclusions that, under the previous conditions, pentobarbital primarily affected control by the keylight rather than the houselight, since when keylights were rendered supplementary, discriminative control of responding was not affected. Further, these results are consistent with the previous results indicating that the effects of pentobarbital on stimulus control depend on the degree of control.

Under the previous conditions, *d*-amphetamine affected stimulus control of behavior only at the highest doses studied. At these doses, disruptions in stimulus control occurred along with pronounced decreases in rates of responding. It might be suggested that the effects of these high doses on stimulus control represent nonspecific alterations in behavior. However, the added discriminative effects of the position of the key attenuated the effects of high doses of *d*-amphetamine suggesting that, even at high doses, specific effects on stimulus control can be detected that might otherwise be overshadowed by marked effects on the output of behavior. Similar types of findings have been reported previously for the disruptions in control of complex sequences of behavior by drugs and toxicants (e.g., Laties, 1972; Laties & Evans, 1980) and might be considered environmental antagonism of a pharmacological effect.

SUMMARY AND IMPLICATIONS

In the present series of studies, discriminative control of responding was established in which the color of the response key on which responses were reinforced was conditional on the status of the houselight stimulus. Under the initial fixed-interval schedule, each response randomly alternated the position of the keylight colors and the houselight was either on or off for the entire fixed interval. With a high degree of stimulus control over responding, none of the drugs studied had appreciable effects on that control across the range of low to intermediate doses that altered rates and patterns of responding. Thus, the effects of the drugs on response rates were not secondary to changes in stimulus control of responding, and it appears that changes in stimulus control of responding contributed little if anything to the changes in rates and patterns of schedule-controlled responding.

Several studies examined the limits to the above findings. For example, pentobarbital, but not any of the other drugs studied, had effects on stimulus control of responding under a discrete-trials procedure. Additionally, when the degree of stimulus control of responding was reduced under the fixed-interval schedule, both pentobarbital and promazine decreased stimulus control at doses that had no effects on the higher levels of stimulus control studied previously, and at doses that were within the range of doses that altered response rates. Thus, the effects of drugs on stimulus control can depend on the conditions under which it is studied. Further, as has been suggested by Dews (1971), the effects of drugs on stimulus control of responding are dependent on the level of stimulus control existing prior to drug administration. Under conditions in which the degree of stimulus control is less than optimal, changes in stimulus control of behavior may contribute to the effects of the drugs on response rates. However, there are levels of stimulus control that are refractory to the effects of drugs, or that are only affected at the highest doses. It is likely that in many of the studies of the effects of drugs on schedule-controlled responding, the levels of stimulus control that exist are refractory to drug-induced change.

Studies of the source of stimulus control disrupted by pentobarbital or d-amphetamine examined the effects of those drugs under the isolated components of the multiple fixed-interval schedule. Under these single-component schedules, the key lights were not conditional discriminative stimuli, and the houselight did not enter into a discriminative role in the prevailing contingencies. However, under the single-component schedules the effects of the drugs on stimulus control of responding were similar to those obtained under the multiple schedule. Therefore, control of behavior by the houselight was not critical for the disruption in stimulus control produced by pentobarbital. Rather, it appears that the discriminative control disrupted by the drug was that exerted by the keylight stimuli.

To further test whether the control of behavior affected by the drugs was primarily that exerted by the color of the keylights, the effects of the drugs were studied under a multiple schedule in which the position of the key colors did not randomly alternate with each response. Under this condition both position and color of the key could serve as discriminative stimuli. At doses of either drug that altered stimulus control under the previous conditions, stimulus control of responding was affected less. Since key color was no longer the sole discriminative stimulus, these results are consistent with the conclusion that the effect on stimulus control under the previous condition was primarily on the control exerted by the keylight colors rather than on the control by the houselight.

With position and key color as redundant discriminative stimuli, A' was greater under control conditions, compared to the previous studies in which the keylight colors alternated with each response. The attenuation of the effects on stimulus control when position was an added discriminative stimulus suggests an environmental antagonism of the drug effect. Operations that increase stimulus control would be expected to attenuate the effects of drugs on stimulus control; conversely, operations that decrease stimulus control would be expected to increase the effects of drugs (e.g., present studies of houselight intensity; see also Witkin, 1986; McKearney, 1970). Obviously, these types of studies are most readily interpreted when there is a method of directly determining the effects of the operations on stimulus control, such as the present measures of A' (see also Moerschbaecher & Thompson, 1980).

Taken together, the results of all of the above studies indicate that the effects of drugs on stimulus control depend most importantly on the degree of control extant prior to drug administration. Further, the results of the studies comparing single component schedules to multiple schedules suggest that the effects depend neither on the conditional nature of the discriminative control, nor on the complexity of the control. Rather, if the conditional nature of the control or the complexity produce a performance that is under relatively less stimulus control, the effects of drugs on that control will be relatively great.

In contrast to the present conclusions, a study by Dews (1955) has been cited to support the notion that the effects of drugs on stimulus control can depend on the complexity, or conditional nature of control. In that study, stimulus control under a conditional discrimination procedure was disrupted by methamphetamine and pentobarbital at doses that did not disrupt the control of performance under "simple" discriminations. However, Dews also found conditions under which stimulus control was disrupted under the "simple" discrimination. Thus, as in the present studies, the critical feature in determining whether stimulus control was disrupted by drugs was not whether the performances were under "simple" or "conditional" stimulus control. In the study by Dews, a higher degree of stimulus control was maintained under the simple discriminations compared to the conditional discrimination. In the present study, a similar level of control was maintained under the two types of discrimination procedures. As Dews (1955) notes, the terms "simple" and "complex" are not easy to define and it is preferable to concentrate on the differential sensitivity of the performances. Since it appears that the differential sensitivity of the performances is related to the nondrug level of stimulus control, it would seem better to concentrate on that feature of the performance than on the operational difference in the schedules. To say that complex discriminations are affected differently from simple discriminations is misleading as it suggests that we know more than we actually do.

Behavioral Mechanisms of Drug Action. The suggestion that drugs can affect stimulus control of behavior implies that drugs can affect behavioral processes as well as behavior itself. As such, effects on behavioral processes can be considered behavioral mechanisms of drug action that underlie the changes in behavior that are observed. Behavioral mechanisms of action were first considered by Dews (1956) when suggesting that the analysis of the behavioral effects of drugs should proceed with a determination of the extent to which the drug effects are like, in the sense of having the same effect on behavior, the effects of the independent variables. For example, a possible mechanism for a drug-induced decrease in rates of responding maintained by food presentation is drug-induced satiety. A drug having this as its exclusive mechanism would have effects on schedule-controlled behavior similar, in all manifestations, to the effects of prefeeding the subject. Thus, an often used method of examining behavioral mechanisms of drug action is the assessment of similarities in performances after drug administration and after some such environmental manipulation (e.g., Dews, 1958; Fig. 2.1). However, the formal equivalence of behavior following a change in an independent variable and administration of a drug can be difficult to directly quantify, and further, can be misleading. For example, as described above, adding a conjunctive fixed-ratio requirement to the fixed-interval schedule had effects on rates and patterns of responding that were similar to those of decreasing the intensity of the houselight. These two operations, however, were functionally different, as was revealed when drugs were administered. There are many examples of formally similar but functionally dissimilar behaviors. Since formal similarity does not imply that the determinants of the behaviors are similar, reliance on formal similarity to infer functional similarity has been termed the Formalistic Fallacy (Skinner, 1969, p. 89f).

Because drugs typically have more than one effect, an effect of the drug occurring along with other effects may not formally resemble the effects of the analogous behavioral modification. Thus, a drug may have an effect through a specific mechanism, as well as other effects on behavior; those other effects may obscure formal equivalence. Therefore formal equivalence should be used only as one preliminary indication of a specific behavioral mechanism of action.

The concept of behavioral mechanism of drug action was expanded though not explicitly defined by Thompson and Schuster (1968) and Laties and Weiss (1969). Each of these publications reviewed several factors that influence the behavioral effects of drugs; however, neither assessed whether the effects of the drugs were similar to the effects of these independent variables. Thompson (1984) more recently defined behavioral mechanism of action as a description of the effects of a drug on a particular behavioral system expressed in terms of some more general set of environmental principles regulating behavior. While this definition is explicit in several respects, it is different from one that requires that the effects of the drug be similar to the effects of some independent variable. Thus, included in Thompson's review of behavioral mechanisms of action are many of the factors that have been shown to influence the behavioral effects of drugs. However, to say that the effects of a drug are *influenced* by, for example, a certain conditioning history of the subject only suggests one factor that may contribute to the behavioral effects of the drug. It does not indicate that the effects of the drug are *similar* to the effects of exposing the subject to that particular history.

As mechanism denotes the primary action of a drug as distinguished from descriptions of resultant effects (Ross & Gilman, 1985), it is appropriate to distinguish between those descriptions indicating that some factor influences the manifestation of a drug action and those descriptions that suggest a manner in which the drugs exert their effects on behavior. Descriptions that indicate only that environmental factors may have an influence on the expression of drug action include factors that are different in kind from those that should be considered mechanisms. The initial suggestion by Dews (1956; see also Dews, 1958, 1970) indicates that the drug effects need be the same as the effects of the independent variable. Rather than require that the effects of the drug and some non-pharmacological (reference) variable be the same, it may be preferable to require that administering the drug and the change in the reference variable be functionally equivalent. A definition requiring functional equivalence is appropriately restrictive, avoids the potentially misleading formal equivalence that may be obtained through different mechanisms, and requires equivalence in the manner in which the drug and some independent variable affect behavior.

One method of determining whether two operations are functionally equivalent is to compare the degree of similarity between the relations of independent and dependent variables. In the case of drug effects, variations in dose can be assessed for similarity to the effects of variations in some dimension of the reference variable. However, any behavioral effects that occur along with the behavioral mechanism of action, would result in functional relations between dose and dependent variable that would not be similar to those obtained between the reference and dependent variables. Assessing the functional equivalence of two nonpharmacological operations may on first blush seem less susceptible to influence by diverse effects of operations. However, different ostensibly equivalent operations have been shown to have varied functional relations to particular behaviors (cf. Miller, 1959). It is likely that most functionally equivalent operations are not singular in their effects, and consequently that functional relations of equivalent operations will more often than not be dissimilar.

In the present studies the effects of drugs on stimulus control were inversely related to the existing level of stimulus control. This result suggested that the drug effect and changes that decrease the degree of stimulus control were functionally equivalent. Another method of assessing functional equivalence is to determine if the effects of the drug are attenuated by an environmental change of the reference variable in the opposite direction of the suggested drug action. This type of result was earlier refered to as an environmental antagonism of drug action. In the present studies, changes that increased stimulus control attenuated the effects of the drugs on that control. Similarly, environmental changes that altered stimulus control in the same direction of the suggested drug action increased the effects of drugs. Assessment of the whether operations interact in this manner appears to be at present the best way to determine whether those operations are functionally equivalent.

ACKNOWLEDGMENTS

Portions of the research described were supported by the following USPHS Grants: DA-02873 awarded to the University of Maryland; DA-00499, MH-02094 and MH-14275 awarded to Harvard Medical School; DA-00254 and DA-03113 awarded to the University of Michigan Medical School; and DA-03505 awarded to the University of Maryland School of Medicine. The work was also supported by USPHS Fellowship DA-01505. The author thanks J. E. Henningfield, R. J. Lamb and J. M. Witkin for comments on the manuscript, and J. E. Barrett for years of advice and support. Technical assistance was provided by W. Abbott, C. Jackson, L. King, F. Adams, R. Rodriguez and S. Fowler. Secretarial help was provided by Mr. T. and C. D. Pro.

REFERENCES

Appel, J. B., Dykstra, L. A. (1977). Drugs, discrimination, and signal detection. In T. Thompson & P. B. Dews (Eds.), *Advances in behavioral pharmacology* (Vol. 1, pp. 139–166). New York: Academic Press.

Berryman, R., Cumming, W. W., Nevin, J. A., & Jarvik, M. E. (1964). Effects of sodium pentobarbital on complex operant discriminations. *Psychopharmacologia, 6,* 388–398.

Boren, M. C. P., & Gollub, L. R. (1972). Accuracy of performance on a matching-to-sample procedure under interval schedules. *Journal of the Experimental Analysis of Behavior, 18,* 65–77.

Dews, P. B. (1955). Studies on behavior. II. The effects of pentobarbital, methamphetamine & scopolamine of performances in pigeons involving discriminations. *Journal of Pharmacology and Experimental Therapeutics, 115,* 380–389.

Dews, P. B. (1956). Modification by drugs of performance on simple schedules of positive reinforcement. *Annals of the New York Academy of Sciences, 65,* 268–281.

Dews, P. B. (1958). Analysis of effects of psychopharmacological agents in behavioral terms. *Federation Proceedings, 17,* 1024–1030.

Dews, P. B. (1970). Drugs in psychology. A commentary on Travis Thompson and Charles R. Schuster's *Behavioral Pharmacology. Journal of the Experimental Analysis of Behavior, 13,* 395–406.

Dews, P. B. (1971). Commentary. In J. A. Harvey (Ed.), *Behavioral analysis of drug action* (pp. 37–43). Glenview, IL: Scott, Foresman.

Dews, P. B., & Morse, W. H. (1961). Behavioral pharmacology. *Annual Review of Pharmacolology, 1,* 145–174.

Dews, P. B., & Wenger G. R. (1977). Rate-dependency of the behavioral effects of amphetamine. In T. Thompson & P. B. Dews (Eds.), *Advances in behavioral pharmacology* (Vol. 1, pp. 167–227). New York: Academic Press.

Dykstra, L. A., & Genovese, R. F. (1987). Measurement of drug effects on stimulus control. In A. J. Greenshaw & C. T. Dourish (Eds.), *Experimental psychopharmacology, concepts and methods* (pp. 393–431). Clifton, NJ: Humana Press.

Ferster, C. B. (1960). Intermittent reinforcement of matching to sample in the pigeon. *Journal of the Experimental Analysis of Behavior, 3,* 259–272.

Ferster, C. B. & Skinner, B. F. (1957). *Schedules of Reinforcement.* New York: Appleton-Century-Crofts.

Green, D. M., & Swets, J. A. (1957). *Signal detection theory and psychophysics.* New York: Wiley.

Grier, J. B. (1971). Nonparametric indexes for sensitivity and bias: Computing formulas. *Psychological Bulletin, 75,* 424–429.

Heise, G. A., & Milar, K. S. (1984). Drugs and stimulus control. In L. L. Iversen, S. D. Iversen & S. H. Snyder (Eds.), *Handbook of psychopharmacology* (Vol. 18, pp. 129–190). New York: Plenum.

Katz, J. L. (1982). Effects of drugs on stimulus control of behavior. I. Independent assessment of effects on response rates and stimulus control. *Journal of Pharmacology and Experimental Therapeutics, 223,* 617–623.

Katz, J. L. (1983). Effects of drugs on stimulus control of behavior. II. Degree of stimulus control as a determinant of effect. *Journal of Pharmacology and Experimental Therapeutics, 226,* 756–763.

Katz, J. L. (1988). Effects of drugs on stimulus control of behavior. III. Analysis of effects of *d*-amphetamine and pentobarbital. *Journal of Pharmacology and Experimental Therapeutics, 246,* 76–83.

Katz, J. L. (1989). Two types of bias in psychophysical detection and recognition procedures: nonparametric indices and effects of drugs. *Psychopharmacology, 97,* 202–205.

Laties, V. G. (1972). The modification of drug effects on behavior by external discriminative stimuli. *Journal of Pharmacology and Experimental Therapeutics, 183,* 1–13.

Laties, V. G. (1975). The role of discriminative stimuli in modulating drug action. *Federation Proceedings, 34,* 1880–1888.

Laties, V. G., & Evans, H. L. (1980). Methylmercury-induced changes in operant discrimination by the pigeon. *Journal of Pharmacology and Experimental Therapeutics, 214,* 620–628.

Laties, V. G., & Weiss, B. (1966). Influence of drugs on behavior controlled by internal and external stimuli. *Journal of Pharmacology and Experimental Therapeutics, 152,* 388–396.

Laties, V. G., & Weiss, B. (1969). Behavioral mechanisms of drug action. In P. Black (Ed.), *Drugs and the brain* (pp. 115–133). Baltimore, MD: The Johns Hopkins Press.

McKearney, J. W. (1970). Rate-dependent effects of drugs: Modification by discriminative stimuli of the effects of amobarbital on schedule-controlled behavior. *Journal of the Experimental Analysis of Behavior, 14,* 167–175.

Miller, N. E. (1959). Liberalization of basic S-R concepts: Extensions to conflict behavior, motivation and social learning. In S. Koch (Ed.), *Psychology: A study of a science* (pp. 196–292). New York: McGraw Hill.

Moerschbaecher, J. M., & Thompson, D. M. (1980). Effects of phencyclidine, pentobarbital, and d-amphetamine on the acquisition and performance of conditional discriminations in monkeys. *Pharmacology Biochemistry and Behavior, 13,* 887–894.

Pollack, I., & Norman, D. A. (1964). A non-parametric analysis of recognition experiments. *Psychonomic Science, 1,* 125–126.

Rees, D. C., Wood, R. W., & Laties, V. G. (1985). The roles of stimulus control and reinforcement frequency in modulating the behavioral effects of d-amphetamine in the rat. *Journal of the Experimental Analysis of Behavior, 43,* 243–255.

Ross, E. M., & Gilman, A. G. (1985). Pharmacodynamics: Mechanisms of drug action and the relationship between drug concetration and effect. In A. G. Gilman, L. S. Goodman, T. Rall, & F. Murad (Eds.), *Goodman and Gilman's The Pharmacological Basis of Therapeutics* (pp. 35–48). New York: Macmillan.

Rutledge, C. O., & Kelleher, R. T. (1965). Interactions between the effects of methamphetamine and pentobarbital on operant behavior in the pigeon. *Psychopharmacologia, 7,* 400–408.

Skinner, B. F. (1969). *Contingencies of reinforcement: A theoretical analysis.* New York: Appleton-Century-Crofts.

Smith, C. B. (1964). Effect of d-amphetamine upon operant behavior of pigeons: enhancement by reserpine. *Journal of Pharmacology and Experimental Therapeutics, 146,* 167–174.

Thompson, D. M. (1978). Stimulus control and drug effects. In D. E. Blackman & D. J. Sanger (Eds.), *Contemporary research in behavioral pharmacology* (pp. 159–207). New York: Plenum Press.

Thompson, T. (1984). Behavioral mechanisms of drug dependence. In T. Thompson, P. B. Dews, & J. E. Barrett (Eds.), *Advances in behavioral pharmacology* (Vol. 4, pp. 1–45). New York: Academic Press.

Thompson, T., & Schuster, C. R. (1968). *Behavioral pharmacology.* Englewood Cliffs, NJ: Prentice Hall.

Witkin, J. M. (1986). Effects of chlorpromazine on fixed-ratio responding: Modification by fixed-interval discriminative stimuli. *Journal of the Experimental Analysis of Behavior, 45,* 195–205.

3 Contributions of the Matching Law to the Analysis of the Behavioral Effects of Drugs

Gene M. Heyman
Harvard University

Michael M. Monaghan
American Cyanamid Company
Lederle Laboratories

INTRODUCTION

William James (1890) used the apt phrase "stream of consciousness" to describe mental life. Had he chosen to describe an organism's overt behavior, he could just as aptly have used the phrase "stream of behavior." For behavior, like consciousness, is continuous, plastic, and reflective of the play of many simultaneously acting forces. Even the task of describing a "simple" organism, such as a rat, engaged in a "simple" task, as pressing a lever, requires that we consider a host of variables, including the response requirement, degree of deprivation, the consequences of lever pressing, and the consequences of engaging in competing activities. Moreover, these variables may interact in complex ways, and historical conditions may matter as well. Faced with this complexity, psychologists have developed techniques for fractionating performance into its component elements. For example, with the method of signal detection (Swets, Tanner, & Birdsall, 1961), it is possible to distinguish changes in perception from changes in motivation. In this chapter we describe a method that decomposes changes in behavior into two components: those that depend on reinforcement processes and those that are a function of motor performance. The method we use is based on the matching law equation (Herrnstein, 1970). Our purpose is to summarize the contribution that this method has made to some long-standing problems in behavioral pharmacology.

THE PROBLEM OF MEASURING A SUBJECT'S SUSCEPTIBILITY TO REINFORCERS

Over the last decade, the interpretation of the effects of antipsychotic drugs on reinforced behavior has been the subject of many research and review papers (e.g., Fibiger, 1978; Wise, 1982). The basic observation is that antipsychotic drugs (often referred to as "neuroleptics") attenuate reinforced responding. For example, they decrease operant responding maintained by the presentation of food and water, and the decreases occur at doses that did not affect food and water intake (compare, e.g., Block & Fisher, 1975; Heyman, 1983; Heyman, Kinzie, & Seiden, 1986; Towell, Muscat, & Willner, 1987; Zis & Fibiger, 1975). The phenomenon has generality, occurring in a wide range of species, including humans (e.g., Fischman & Schuster, 1979), and with a variety of reinforcers, including ones that are not consumed, such a brain stimulation (e.g., Gallistel & Karras, 1984). However, the behavioral mechanisms mediating the effects of neuroleptics on reinforced behavior have not been clearly established.

Some evidence suggests that neuroleptics attenuate reinforcement processes. For example, in a threshold prodcedure in which the reinforcer was brain stimulation and the subjects were rats (Zarevics & Setler, 1979), pimozide, a neuroleptic, increased the threshold. That is, the subjects had the capacity to respond, but required a higher level of reinforcement to do so. However, other results appear to contradict the reinforcement interpretation and suggest instead that neuroleptics produce a motor deficit. For example, Ettenberg, Koob, and Bloom (1981) showed that a neuroleptic induced decrease in reinforced responding depended on the response requirement. A 0.1 mg/kg dose of alpha-flupentixol reduced reinforced lever pressing by about 35% but had no effect on reinforced nose-poking. This suggests that alpha-flupentixol affected the capacity to respond and therefore the more effortful response was differentially affected.

These apparently conflicting findings stimulated attempts to experimentally dissociate reinforcement efficacy and motor performance. However, despite numerous studies, the controversy persisted (see, for example, Wise, 1982, and accompanying commentary). The problem has been in part methodological. Most results could be interpreted in at least two ways. For example, consider a study that is frequently cited as showing a neuroleptic-induced reinforcement deficit.Wise, Spindler, deWit and Gerber (1978) compared the effects of pimozide and extinction (removing the reinforcer) on response rate. Rats served as subjects, and in baseline conditions, each response (a lever press) was reinforced. Pimozide and extinction produced similar patterns of response rate decline. At the beginning of the session, response rates were at baseline levels and, then, with time, gradually subsided. Wise et al. (1978) explained the pimozide effect as a drug induced attenuation of reinforcement. They reasoned that pimozide affected reinforcement process and not motor performance, because its effects were similar to those that follow removing the reinforcer. However, the results are also compatible with the view that pimozide produced a motor deficit. In the Wise et al. study, reinforcement rate was proportional to response rate. Thus if a motor impairment slowed response rate, it would also reduce reinforcement rate. The decrease in reinforcement rate would in turn decrease response rate, and, because of this positive feed-back loop, response and reinforcement rate would gradually decline, just as in extinction. In support of this motor interpretation, pimozide does not produce an extinction-like pattern of response rate decline in procedures which do not maintain a proportionality between response and reinforcement rates (e.g., Fibiger, Carter, & Phillips, 1976).

The extinction procedure for measuring reinforcement efficacy thus seems ambiguous, and in other studies researchers found that neuroleptics changed response rates in ways not observed during extinction (Gramling, Fowler, & Collins, 1984). In contrast, the matching law equation, as we hope to show, leads to measures of reinforcement efficacy and motor performance that are logically independent and have been empirically validated. The results displayed in Fig. 3.1 (Heyman & Monaghan, 1987) introduce the matching law approach.

THE MATCHING LAW EQUATION: BASIC FINDINGS

The top left panel shows the effects of deprivation on response rate. The subjects were 8 water deprived rats, the response requirement was a lever press, and the reinforcer was a small portion of water (0.025 ml). The basic reinforcement contingency was set by a variable-interval schedule, which intermittently reinforced lever press responses according to the passage of time. Each session consisted of a series of five variable-interval reinforcement schedules, and each schedule was available for 9 min with a 5 min time-out period between reinforcement schedules. The mean programmed reinforcement times ranged from 150 sec (25 reinforcers per hour) to 5 sec (720 reinforcers per hour). The two deprivation periods were 6.0 and 47.5 hours.

Response rate was a negatively accelerated function of reinforcement rate, and, relatedly, at the two highest reinforcement rates (approximately 340 and 700 per hour), response rates were similar, especially in the extended deprivation period (47.5 hours). In other words, there was a response rate ceiling, as indeed there must be, so that once responding approached this level, further increases in reinforcement rate had little effect on response rate. The horizontal dashed lines are an estimate of the response rate asymptotes for the two conditions (an explanation of how this limit was estimated is offered in the description of the matching law equation).

Deprivation increased response rates, and the increases were an inverse function of reinforcement rate. Or, in terms of the estimated response rate asymptotes, deprivation increased the rate at which response rates approached their

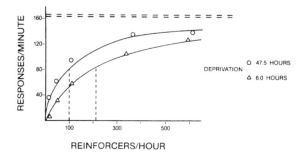

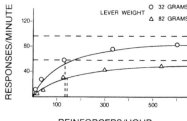

REINFORCERS/HOUR

FIG. 3.1. The effect of water deprivation and lever weight on reinforced responding. The open symbols represent group median results
(Heyman & Monaghan, 1987). The curves show the predicted relationship between response rate and reinforcement rate, according to
the matching law equation. The horizontal dashed lines indicate the
response rate asymptotes (k), and the vertical dashed lines represent
the rate of reinforcement that maintained a one-half asymptotic response rate (R_e).

asymptote. This effect was conveniently shown by the two vertical dashed lines.
They mark the rates of reinforcement that maintained a one-half asymptotic
response rate. For example, in the high deprivation condition, 100 reinforce-
ments per hour maintained a one-half asymptotic response rate, but in the low
deprivation condition, a rate of about 220 reinforcers an hour was needed to
maintain a one-half asymptotic response rate. Thus for the longer deprivation
condition, water was a more potent or efficacious reinforcer. This finding suggests that the rate of reinforcement for a one-half asymptotic response rate can be
used to measure reinforcement efficacy.

   The lower right panel of Fig. 3.1 shows the results from a study in which the
weight of the lever was varied. The deprivation period was fixed at 23.5 hours
and the response requirement was varied, but otherwise the procedure was identical to that used in the previous study (including the same 8 rats). Changes in the

response requirement produced a different pattern of response rate shifts than did changes in deprivation. As the horizontal dashed lines indicate, there was a shift in the estimated response rate asymptote, whereas the rate of reinforcement for a one-half asymptotic response rate remained about the same (the vertical dashed lines). Other researchers have shown that increases in the weight of the manipulandum increased response duration (see Fowler, Gramling, & Liao, 1986). Consequently, it is likely that the decrease in response rate asymptote was due to an increase in response duration. In any case, the study suggests that the response rate asymptote can be used to measure the effects of treatments that affect motor performance.

The Matching Law Equation

The smooth curves and dashed lines in Fig. 3.1 were obtained by fitting the matching law equation to the data sets. The customary notation is:

$$B = \frac{k\,R}{R + R_e},$$ (1)

where B represents response rate, R represents reinforcement rate, and k and R_e are fitted parameters. Figure 3.2 shows the equation along with the parameter

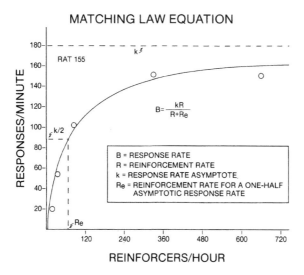

FIG. 3.2. The matching law equation and representative results (Heyman & Monaghan, 1987). The open circles show the average response rates.

definitions and a data set from our laboratory. The magnitude of k is equal to the estimated asymptotic response rate (note that response rate approaches but does not exceed k as reinforcement rate is increased). Thus the horizontal dashed lines in Figs. 3.1 and 3.2 were obtained by fitting the matching law equation to the data sets and finding the values for k. For example, in the deprivation study summarized in Fig. 3.1, the estimated values of k were 170 and 166 responses per min (k is measured in the same units as is the dependent variable, e.g., responses per minute). The parameter R_e is equal to the rate of reinforcement that maintains a one-half asymptotic response rate ($B = k/2$ when $R = R_e$). Thus the vertical dashed lines in Figs. 3.1 and 3.2 were determined by fitting the matching law equation to the data and finding the value of R_e. For example, in the lever weight experiment (Fig. 3.1), the estimated values of R_e were 143 and 147 reinforcers per hour (R_e is measured in the same units as is the independent variable, e.g., reinforcers per hour). Equation 1, then, says that response rate is a function of three variables: reinforcement rate, the determinants of the asymptote (k), and the determinants of the rate of reinforcement that maintains a one-half asymptotic response rate (R_e).

The matching law equation accounted for over 90% of the variance in response rates for the results displayed in Fig. 3.1. Similar results have been obtained with different species, including humans, with different reinforcers, including ones that are not consumed, such as brain stimulation, and with different response requirements, for example, running, lever pressing, and swimming. (For a review of the matching law literature see de Villiers & Herrnstein, 1976.) Thus the matching law equation provides a quantitative and general account of the relationship between response rate and reinforcement rate.

Experimental Manipulations that Affect the Matching Law Parameters

Figure 3.1 suggests that the matching law equation can be used to evaluate the effects of drugs on motor performance and reinforcement efficacy. We reviewed the literature to determine the generality of this conclusion. The review was restricted to studies in which the parameter estimates were based on at least 5 data points and in which the response was maintained by a positive reinforcer.

There were four experiments in which k systematically changed and R_e did not (see Heyman & Monaghan, 1987 for references). In each one, the experimenter varied the response requirement. For example, in a study in which the subjects were pigeons, the manipulandum was varied: a button, which the pigeons pecked, was replaced with a treadle, which they kicked (McSweeney, 1978). The primary result was a 60% decrease in k. In contrast, changes in R_e were small and non-systematic. Changes in the response requirement alter the topography of the response, for example, its duration, and also, perhaps, affect the subject's capacity to respond. In addition to these empirical results, derivations of the matching law equation (Herrnstein, 1974, 1979; Heyman, 1988) support the conclusion that k measures motor performance. Thus both empirical and logical considerations lead to the conclusion that k is a measure of motor performance.

There are 10 studies in which R_e systematically varied but k did not. The experimental manipulations included changes in reward magnitude, reward quality, and deprivation (see Heyman & Monaghan, 1987, for references). Thus changes in the conditions of reinforcement altered R_e, with increases in reward magnitude and deprivation period producing decreases in R_e. For example, in a study with rats in which the reinforcer was brain stimulation (Hamilton, Stellar, & Hart, 1985), increases in current intensity decreased R_e without affecting k. (The more potent the reinforcer, the less needed to maintain a one-half asymptotic response rate.) In addition to the empirical studies, the previously mentioned derivations of the matching law equation (Herrnstein, 1974, 1979; Heyman, 1988) implied that R_e was a function of the relative reinforcing efficacy of the reinforcer maintaining the response. Thus there is both empirical and logical support for the conclusion that R_e provides a measure of the efficacy of the reinforcer maintaining the measured response.

There are also several studies in which a change in the reinforcement conditions affected both k and R_e (e.g., Bradshaw, Szabadi, & Bevan, 1978; Snyderman, 1983). This result is not necessarily discrepant with a change in just R_e. For example, rats do not lever press in the same way for food and water reinforcers (e.g., Davey & Cleland, 1982; Hull, 1977), so that a change from water to food reinforcement should affect both k and R_e. However, the experiments in which both k and R_e changed were similar to ones in which just R_e had changed. For example, in four studies, differences in deprivation produced systematic differences in R_e but not k. (Bradshaw, Szabadi, Ruddle, & Pears, Conrad & Sidman, 1956; Heyman & Monaghan, 1987; Logan, 1960). In contrast, Snyderman (1983) found that changes in deprivation affected both k and R_e. This apparent discrepancy may be due to factors other than deprivation. For example, in the Snyderman experiment, the richest reinforcement component typically did not maintain the highest response rate. This may have occurred because the subjects had either partially satiated and/or were not given sufficient time to consume the reinforcer (see Heyman & Monaghan, 1987, for details). Moreover, it the data are analyzed without the non-monotonic data point, the results show a systematic relationship between deprivation and R_e and little change in k, just as in the other deprivation studies (Heyman, 1988). Thus the simplest account of the literature is that k measures motor performance, R_e measures reinforcement efficacy, and, in addition, there are a number of experiments in which changes in reinforcement conditions were associated with changes in k because of uncontrolled factors. Importantly, that k and R_e can vary independently does not deny that certain, more complex, manipulations will systematically alter both parameters.

NEUROLEPTICS

Next we describe studies in which the matching law equation was used to analyze the effects of neuroleptics on reinforced responding. A change in the rate of reinforcement that maintained a one-half asymptotic response rate was used to measure reinforcement effects. Throughout this chapter this measure is referred to as "reinforcement efficacy" or "susceptibility to reinforcement." When it changes, a given rate of reinforcement maintains more or less responding relative to the subject's asymptotic response rate. Change in the asymptotic response rate was used to measure motor performance. As noted in the discussion of Figs. 3.1 and 3.2 this measure varies systematically with changes in the response requirement.

The procedure for the neuroleptic studies was similar to the deprivation and lever weight studies summarized in Fig. 3.1. Rats served as subjects (6 to 8 per experiment). They were water deprived for 23.5 hours, and the reinforcer was a small portion of water (0.025 ml). Sessions were divided into five reinforcement periods. Each period provided a different reinforcement rate, with a range of about 20 to 700 reinforcers per hour, and each period was available for 7 to 9 min depending on the study. The five different reinforcement rates were distinguished by combinations of auditory and visual stimuli, and the order was random, without replacement. A time-out period separated reinforcement components; its duration was 5 to 9 min, depending on the study.

The drugs tested were: chlorpromazine, pimozide, fluphenazine decanoate, and cis-flupentixol. Chlorpromazine, pimozide, and cis-flupentixol were administered acutely, either once or twice per week. The acute injections were at a concentration of 1 ml per kilogram and were delivered intraperitoneally. Each dose was given three times, and vehicle injections were interspersed between drug doses.

Drug effects were described in terms of changes in response rate and changes in the matching law parameters. The parameters were obtained from each subject in each condition. These quantities were then subjected to either paired t tests or analysis of variance to determine statistical significance. A weighted least squares technique was used to fit the equation and estimate the parameters (Wilkinson, 1960). The method is based on the fact that the reciprocal transformation of the matching law equation is linear: $1/B = 1/k + R_e/kR_e$. The sample sizes for the fitting procedure were three sessions for acute drug conditions, 6 sessions for chronic drug conditions, and typically 10 or more sessions for baseline and vehicle conditions.

Chlorpromazine and Pimozide

Figures 3.3, 3.4, and 3.5 show the effects of pimozide and chlorpromazine on response rate. The changes were dose dependent, and individual subject response rates (Figs. 3.3 and 3.4) were similar to group median response rates (Fig. 3.5).

46

INDIVIDUAL SUBJECT RESPONSE RATE: PIMOZIDE

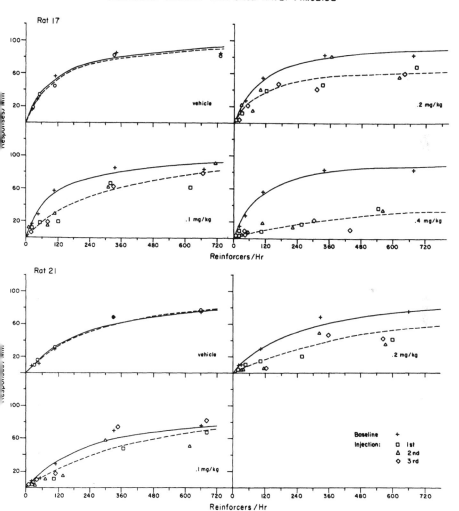

FIG. 3.3.   The effect of pimozide on reinforced responding for two representative subjects. The open symbols show the response rates for each of the three sessions that each dose was administered. The crosses show the average response rates in baseline.

INDIVIDUAL SUBJECT RESPONSE RATE: CHLORPROMAZINE

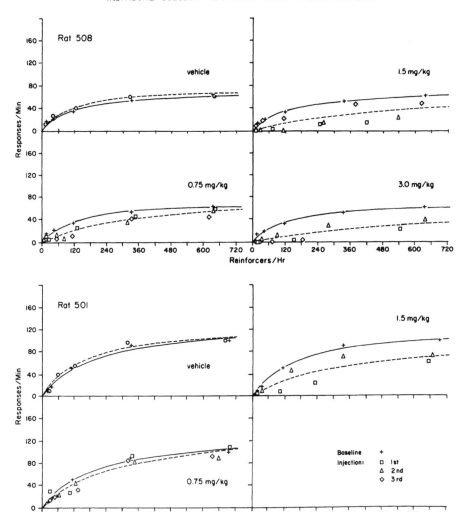

FIG. 3.4. The effect of chlorpromazine on reinforced responding. The format is the same as in Fig. 3.3.

GROUP MEDIAN RESPONSE RATES:

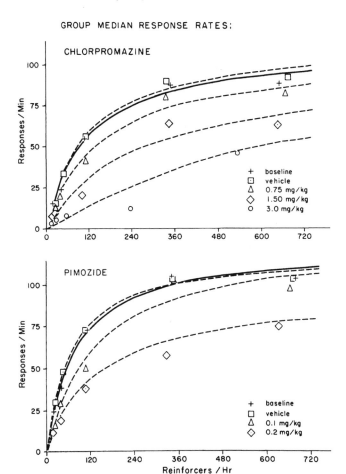

FIG. 3.5. The median response rates in the pimozide and chlorpromazine experiments.

The lowest dose of pimozide (0.1 mg/kg) and chlorpromazine (0.75 mg/kg) decreased response rates maintained by the lower reinforcement rates, but had little or no effect on response rates maintained by the highest reinforcement rate (VI 5 sec schedule). For example, drug session response rates for Rat 17 at the 0.1 mg/kg dose of pimozide (open symbols in Fig. 3.3) were invariably lower than baseline session response rates (crosses) in the four lowest reinforcement rate components. In contrast, drug session response rates overlapped baseline session response rates in the richest reinforcement rate component (VI 5 sec schedule). However, at higher doses, chlorpromazine and pimozide decreased response rates in all five reinforcement rate components. For example, drug session response rates for Rat 17 at the two higher pimozide doses (0.2 and 0.4 mg/kg) were invariably lower than baseline response rates. (Rat 17 was atypical in that it continued to respond at the 0.4 mg/kg dose.)

The 0.1 mg/kg dose of pimozide and 0.75 mg/kg dose of chlorpromazine produced response rate changes that were similar to those that occurred in studies in which the deprivation period or amount of reinforcement was decreased (see Fig. 3.1; Heyman & Monaghan, 1987). Thus at these doses, pimozide and chlorpromazine decreased reinforcement efficacy independently of changes in motor performance. However, at higher doses the pattern of response rate change was more complex, resembling the combined effects of changes in the response requirement and reinforcement conditions.

Figure 3.6 shows that chlorpromazine and pimozide produced dose dependent increases in R_e. The changes were large, with 7 of 8 subjects showing an increase at the lowest chlorpromazine dose and 7 of 7 showing an increase at the lowest pimozide dose. Changes in k were also dose dependent, but at the lowest dose neither pimozide nor chlorpromazine systematically affected k. Thus, according to the matching law equation criteria, these two neuroleptics decreased reinforced reponding in two different ways: they reduced reinforcement efficacy and reduced motor performance.

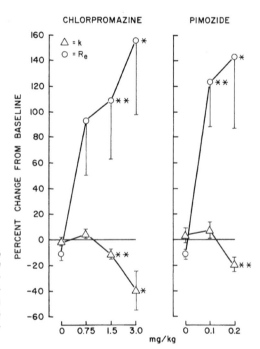

FIG. 3.6. Changes in k and R_e as a function of drug dose. The open symbols depict the average percent change from baseline. A single asterik indicates a significance level of .05 and two asteriks indicate a .01 level, according to a paired t test.

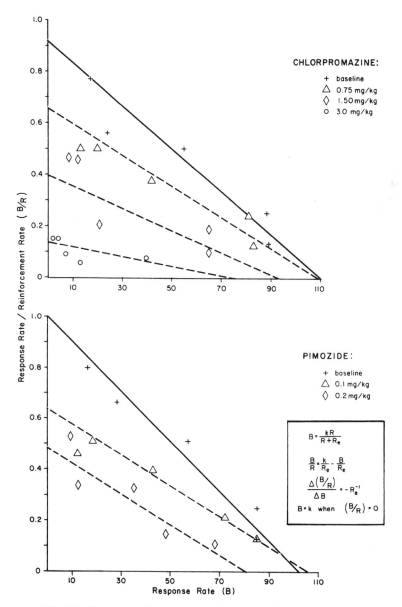

FIG. 3.7. Scatchard plot of the effects of chlorpromazine and pimozide on response rate. This graph is based on analogies between receptor binding and reinforced behavior (Heyman, 1988). A decrease in the slope is equivalent to a decrease in reinforcement efficacy and a leftward shift in the x-axis intercept is equivalent to motor slowing.

Figure 3.7 shows another way of displaying matching law analyses of changes in reinforced responding. The graph was adapted from a Scatchard (1949) plot of receptor binding. The data can be displayed in this way because the matching law equation has the same form as the basic equation used to describe the relationship between concentration of ligand and concentration of bound receptors (see, e.g., Clark, 1933). The analogous independent variables are reinforcement rate and ligand concentration and the analogous dependent variables are response rate and bound receptor concentration. (The relationship between the matching law equation and receptor binding equation is described in more detail elsewhere; see Heyman, 1988). In order to display the data as in Fig. 3.7, the matching law equation was rearranged so that: $B/R = (k\text{-}B)/R_e$. In this form there is a linear relationship between B/R and B, and the resulting line has a slope of $-1/R_e$ and intersects the x-axis at k. Thus, decrease in slope indicates a decrease in reinforcement efficacy, and a leftward shift in the x-axis intersection indicates a decrease in motor performance.

Fluphenazine Decanoate

Pimozide and chlorpromazine were administered once or twice a week, and their effects could be measured in hours. In contrast, psychiatric patients are dosed daily or are given long lasting depot injections. We attempted to mimic the clinical dosing regime by giving the rats intramuscular injections of a neuroleptic-lipid mixture: fluphenazine decanoate. The lipid slowly breaks down, thereby releasing the fluphenazine. The release rate is very gradual. For example, in a study with humans the drug was detected as long as 6 months after administration (Wistedt, Jorgensen, & Wiles, 1982).

Figures 3.8 and 3.9 show the effect of fluphenazine decanoate on k and R_e as a function of time since injection. The points represent the median subject value, using blocks of six consecutive sessions as the samples (in the acute studies, three sessions were used). In that there were 6 subjects in the 2.50 mg/kg group and 8 in the 5.0 mg/kg group, the data points represent 36 and 48 sessions respectively.

The 2.5 and 5.0 doses increased R_e and decreased k, just as did higher doses of pimozide and chlorpromazine. The magnitude and duration of the changes were dose dependent. The effects of the 2.5 mg/kg dose persisted for about 30 to 40 sessions, and at the 5.0 mg/kg dose, the return to baseline took about 90 sessions for k and about 54 sessions for R_e. Put somewhat differently, the mass of data summarized in Figs. 3.8 and 3.9 underscores the point that widely used neuroleptics decrease both reinforcement efficacy and motor performance. The data in Fig. 3.8 (changes in k) also suggest that chronic fluphenazine decanoate may have produced irreversible motor effects. For 11 of 14 subjects (both groups), k recovered to higher than baseline levels. This overshot could have been due to chronic drug treatment or, of course, age related changes (the rats were approximately five months old when drug treatment began).

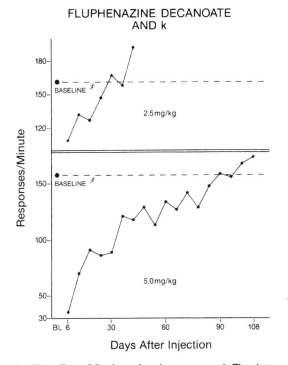

FIG. 3.8.   The effect of fluphenazine decanoate on k. The data points show the group medians, as calculated from samples of six consecutive sessions.

Cis-flupentixol

Cis-flupentixol is derived from phenothiazine and, accordingly, is structurally similar to chlorpromozine (see, e.g., Baldesarrini, 1980). It is referred to as a neuroleptic and shares a number of the defining characteristics of this class of drugs. It is an effective antipsychotic (Stauning, Kirk, & Jorgensen, 1979), it attenuates reinforced responding (e.g., Hamilton et al., 1985), and it antagonizes the behavioral effects of dopamine agonists (e.g., Herrera-Marschitz & Ungerstedt, 1984). However, unlike chlorpromazine, pimozide, and fluphenazine decanoate, cis-flupentixol decreased reinforced responding at doses that did not decrease reinforcement efficacy. Two studies showed this result.

Heyman, Monaghan, and Clody (1987) evaluated the effects of cis-flupentixol on k and R_e in a study in which the procedure was identical to that used in the pimozide and chlorpromazine experiments. The subjects were 8 rats, the reinforcer was water, and the response requirement was a lever press. Figures 3.10, 3.11, and 3.12 show the results. Cis-flupentixol produced dose dependent de-

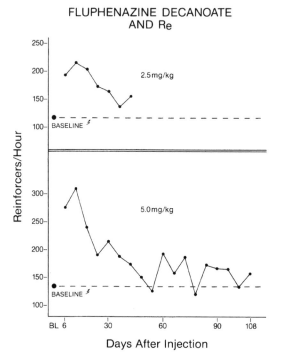

FLUPHENAZINE DECANOATE
AND Re

FIG. 3.9.   The effect of fluphenazine decanoate on R_e. The format is the same as in Fig. 3.8.

creases in k (Fig. 3.11). In contrast, changes R_e were not systematic (Fig. 3.12), although at the two lowest doses (.005 and .01 mg/kg) there was the suggestion of a decrease in R_e and there was an overall increase in the variability of R_e, which was not dose dependent. Hamilton et al., (1985) obtained similar results. The reinforcer in their study was brain stimulation, but otherwise their procedure was like the ones described in this chapter. They tested three subjects and found dose dependent decreases in k for two (.05 to .20 mg/kg), whereas the changes in R_e were not systematic. Thus cis-flupentixol, unlike the other neuroleptics that we evaluated, reduced motor performance at doses that did not reduce reinforcement efficacy.

The matching law analysis distinguished cis-flupentixol from other neuroleptics. Biochemical and clinical criteria also distinguish cis-flupentixol. Cis-flupentixol is a mixed D1-D2 antagonist. Its affinity for D2 sites is within the range set by pimozide and chlorpromazine (Hyttel & Arnt, 1986). However, its affinity for D1 sites is quite different. Cis-flupentixol's affinity for D1 sites is more than 15 times greater than that of chlorpromazine and about 100 times greater than that of pimozide (Hyttel & Arnt, 1986). Fluphenazine is similar to pimozide and chlorpromazine in that it has a higher affinity for D2 sites than for D1 sites. Thus cis-flupentixol's effect on motor performance may be related to its capacity to bind about equally well to D1 and D2 sites and/or its relative high affinity for D1 sites. The receptor affinity findings also suggest that chlorpromazine and pimozide's effect on reinforcement efficacy may be related to the difference in their affinities for D1 and D2 sites, namely that they have a higher affinity for D2 receptors.

Cis-flupentixol is used in the treatment of schizophrenia and schizoaffective disorder (Parent & Toussaint, 1983; Singh, 1984). According to clinical impres-

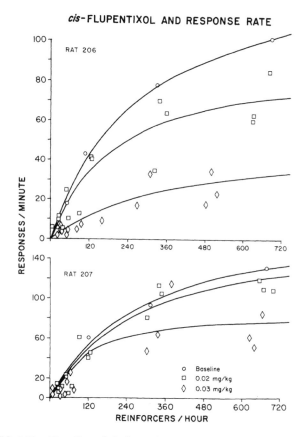

FIG. 3.10.   The effect of cis-flupentixol on reinforced responding. The open squares and diamonds show the response rates for the three sessions that each dose was administered. The open circles show the average baseline response rates.

cis - FLUPENTIXOL AND k

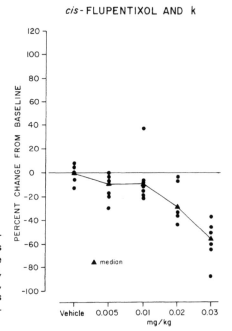

FIG. 3.11.   The effect of cis-flu-pentixol on k. Each point shows the percentage change for one of the 8 subjects. (However, there are not always 8 points, because some subjects' scores were too close together to represent with two points.)

sions and data collected using the Brief Psychiatric Rating Scale (BPRS), it is more likely to reduce depression and anxiety than the other neuroleptics with which it has been compared. For example, Singh (1984) observed that cis-flupentixol reduced depression, whereas other neuroleptics produce dysphoria; Parent and Toussaint reported that cis-flupentixol produced a significant decrease on the depression-anxiety subscale of the BPRS, whereas haloperidol did not.

Although we have tested just four neuroleptics, the available results show a correlation between change in R_e and changes in mood: Chlorpromazine, pimozide, and fluphenazine decanoate increased R_e and are reported to produce dysphoria; cis-flupentixol is said not to produce dysphoria and did not increase R_e.

Summary of Neuroleptic Results

Other researchers have used the matching law or similar methods to analyze the behavioral effects of neuroleptics. Although procedures varied from laboratory to laboratory, the results were similar. In a study in which the subjects were food deprived rats and the reinforcer was a small portion of milk (Heyman, 1983), pimozide increased R_e and decreased k, just as in experiments in which the subjects were water deprived. Similar results were obtained in a study with nondeprived rats (Hamilton et al., 1985). The procedure was a five component multiple schedule, as in the studies discussed earlier, but the reinforcer was brain stimulation. Pimozide increased R_e and decreased k_e just as in experiments in which the subjects were food and water deprived. Thus pimozide produced the same pattern of changes in the matching law parameters independently of the subject's deprivation state and the type of reinforcer. Gallistel and his colleagues (e.g., Gallistel, Shizgal, & Yeomans, 1981) developed a method for distinguishing between changes in motor performance and reinforcement efficacy that is similar to the matching law approach. In their experiments rats were used as subjects and brain stimulation was the reinforcer. In each session a dimension of brain stimulation was varied (e.g., current intensity), and the experimenters estimated the subject's asymptotic response level and the reinforcement setting that maintained a one-half asymptotic response level. Gallistel estimated these parameters by eye, however de Villiers and Herrnstein (1976) showed that the matching law equation described Gallistel's results.

In the brain-stimulation reward studies (Gallistel & Davis, 1983; Gallistel & Karras, 1984) chlorpromazine and pimozide decreased reinforcement efficacy. There were no apparent changes in motor performance, so that changes in reinforcement efficacy had a lower dose threshold, as in the water deprivation studies. Franklin (1978) used Gallistel's approach to evaluate the effects of pimozide on reinforced behavior in a runway apparatus. The rat was placed in a start box and then given a brief pulse of brain stimulation upon reaching the end of the alley. Pimozide increased the current intensity required to maintain a one-

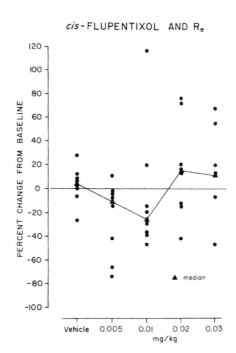

FIG. 3.12. The effect of cis-flupentixol on R_e. The format is
the same as in Fig. 3.11.

half asymptotic running speed, and did so at doses that did not reduce the estimated asymptotic running speed. Thus the results from several laboratories indicate that pimozide and chlorpromazine reduced both reinforcement efficacy and motor performance and that the dose threshold for the reinforcement effects was lower. More generally the findings suggest that the pharmacology of reinforcement processes has core elements that are common to a number, perhaps all, reinforcers.

In contrast to the results just reviewed, Morley, Bradshaw, and Szabadi (1984) concluded that pimozide slowed motor performance at doses that did not affect reinforcement efficacy. Their evidence is the pattern of response rate changes in two different variable-interval schedules. One schedule provided a relatively high reinforcement rate (VI 10 sec), the other a relatively low rate (VI 100 sec). Each schedule was run separately, and the VI 10-sec schedule was in effect first. As there were just two reinforcement schedules, it was not possible to estimate k and R_e. However, Morley et al. pointed out that it is possible to infer how these parameters behaved. Proportional shifts in response rate imply that k changed and larger response rate shifts in the low reinforcement rate schedule imply that R_e changed. Pimozide (.125 to .5 mg/kg) reduced response rates, but at some doses the decreases were larger on the VI 10 sec schedule and at other doses the decreases were larger on the VI 100 sec schedule, so that there was no difference as a function of reinforcement rate. Morley et al. concluded that pimozide reduced motor performance. However, inferences about motor performance and reinforcement efficacy that are based on the performance in just two conditions may be ambiguous. One of the problems is the following.

Morley et al. used dose levels that in the 5-condition procedures produce both motor and reinforcement effects. However, Morley et al. did not test whether their procedure would detect changes in reinforcement efficacy if changes in motor performance also occurred, and, more generally, validation studies were not conducted. Possibly, then, Morley et al.'s results are not discrepant, but simply ambiguous because the procedure under certain conditions is not sensitive to changes in reinforcement efficacy. In any case, in experiments in which the researchers employed enough conditions to estimate the matching law parameters, pimozide has affected the reinforcement efficacy parameter. (Franklin, 1978; Gallistel & Karras, 1984; Hamilton et al., 1985; Heyman, 1983; Heyman et al., 1986).

AMPHETAMINE

Several lines of evidence indicate that neuroleptic behavioral effects are mediated in a significant way by the neurotransmitter dopamine. In vitro studies show that neuroleptics block dopamine postsynaptic receptor sites and that their affinity for such sites typically is higher than for other sites (e.g., Creese, 1983). Patients receiving neuroleptics often show parkinsonian symptoms, and postmortem evaluations indicate that parkinson's patients suffered from a depletion of dopamine cells in the neostriatum (e.g., Iversen & Iversen, 1975). Consequently, it is plausible that the neuroleptic-induced changes in k and R_e were mediated by dopamine receptors. This hypothesis was tested by evaluating the effects of amphetamine on the matching law parameters. Amphetamine increases the availability of dopamine at postsynaptic receptor sites (e.g., Cooper, Bloom, & Roth, 1986). Thus if dopamine mediates changes in k and R_e, amphetamine, especially at low doses, should increase k and decrease R_e. A matching law analysis of amphetamine was also of interest because of previous interpretations of its behavioral effects. According to some researchers, amphetamine-induced changes in response rate are mediated by changes in reinforcement processes, whereas others attribute the response rate effects to changes in motor performance. For example, Berlyne, Koenig, and Hirota (1966) suggested that low doses of amphetamine increased reinforcement efficacy and high doses decreased it, but Lyon and Robbins assumed that amphetamine's primary behavioral effect is to alter response topography, and, in support of this view, Fowler, Filewich, and Leberer (1977) showed that amphetamine increased response force at doses of 0.8 and 1.6 mg/kg. Thus, as with neuroleptics, the interpretation of the behavioral changes was uncertain.

Changes in Response Rate and Matching Law Parameters

The procedure for the amphetamine experiment was virtually the same as the one for the pimozide, chlorpromazine, and cis-flupentixol studies. The subjects were rats, the reinforcer was water, and five different reinforcement rates were presented in random order, with a range of about 20 to 700 per hour. Figure 3.13 shows that under these conditions, 0.25 to 1.0 mg/kg doses of amphetamine typically increased response rates, with relatively larger increases at the lower reinforcement rates. In contrast, the 2.0 mg/kg dose increased response rate only at the highest reinforcement rate, and the 3.0 mg/kg decreased response rate at all reinforcement rates. Figure 3.14 shows that changes in R_e were bitonic. Low doses decreased R_e and high doses increased it. The average change in k was monotonically increasing (but see individual results below). The 2.0 mg/kg dose produced a significant increase, but the 3.0 mg/kg dose did not because of subject variability (see below). Thus the changes in reinforcement efficacy followed the pattern predicted by Berlyne et al. (1966): Low doses increased reinforcement efficacy and high doses decreased it. However, there were also changes in motor performance as suggested by Lyon and Robbins (1975). There was a dose dependent increase in the average response rate asymptote.

GROUP AVERAGE RESPONSE RATE

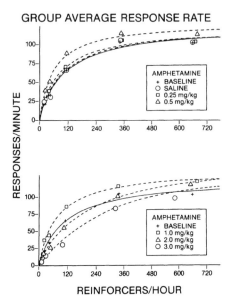

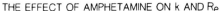

FIG. 3.13. The effect of amphetamine on reinforced responding. The data points show the group average response rates. The curves show the matching law equation predictions of the relationship between response rate and reinforcement rate.

REINFORCERS/HOUR

THE EFFECT OF AMPHETAMINE ON k AND R$_e$

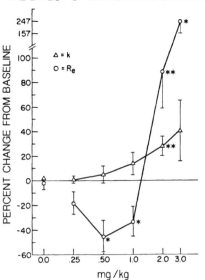

FIG. 3.14. The effect of amphetamine on k and R_e. The open symbols show the average percentage change from baseline. A single asterik indicates a significance level of .05, and two asteriks indicate a .01 level, according to a paired t test.

Individual Differences

Group measures, such as the averages displayed in Fig. 3.14 can reveal general trends. However, averaging can also hide orderly relations if the dependent measure is a nonmonotonic function of the independent variable and individuals differ in terms of their sensitivity to the independent variable. Under these circumstances normalizing the results reveals patterns that would be obscured by averaging. Figure 3.15 provides an example. On the y-axis is change in k and on the x-axis is drug dose as a function of the dose that produced the largest increase (noted as "peak"). For example, for one subject the 3.0 dose produced the largest increase in k, so that the peak-1 dose is 2.0, whereas for another subject, the 1.0 dose produced the largest change so that the peak-1 dose is 0.5 mg/kg. When the results are arranged in this manner, changes in k are bitonic, just as they were for R_e. This pattern is consisted with the findings of other researchers. Bradshaw, Ruddle, and Szabadi (1981) found that amphetamine (0.6 mg/kg) decreased k, and, more generally, high doses of amphetamine typically decrease reinforced responding (e.g., Lyon & Robbins, 1975).

The results from the amphetamine study support the hypothesis that dopamine mediates changes in reinforcement efficacy and/or motor performance. Neu-

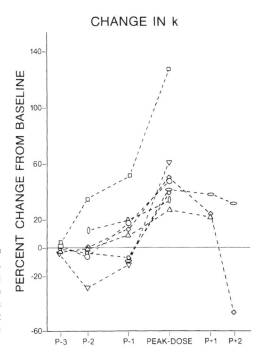

FIG. 3.15. The effects of amphetamine on k, using a normalized x-axis. Each symbol shows the results for one of the 8 subjects, and the x-axis shows dose relative to the one that produced the largest increase in k (see text).

roleptics and amphetamine have opposite effects on the availability of dopamine and they had opposite effects on the matching law parameters. However, the relationships between dopamine and reinforcement efficacy and/or motor performance may be quite complex, since changes in k and R_e were nonmonotonic.

Rate Dependency Principle: A Reinterpretation

We have described the effects of amphetamine on reinforced responding in terms of three variables: reinforcement rate, reinforcement efficacy, and motor performance. An alternative approach is available. In behavioral pharmacology, the effects of amphetamine on reinforced responding are usually described as "rate dependent." This principle, introduced by Dews (e.g., 1958), states that the magnitude of a drug induced change in behavior depends on that behavior's baseline level. For example, if we had presented a rate dependent analysis, the baseline level of responding would have been treated as an independent variable, and it, rather than reinforcement rate, would have been plotted along the x-axes of the graphs. Response based analyses have figured largely in behavioral pharmacology: In scores of studies drug effects have been plotted as a function of baseline response rate (e.g., Dews & Wenger, 1977; Kelleher & Morse, 1968); Robbins (1981) described the principle as one of behavioral pharmacology's two most important contributions to the study of behavior; and Pickens (1977), in his history of behavioral pharmacology, listed rate dependency as one of three major approaches to the study of the behavioral effects of drugs. But according to the matching law equation, response rate is a dependent variable. Consequently, if both the matching law equation and the rate dependency principle can describe the same set of results, it should be possible to establish the logical relationships between the two and, also, determine which provides the more accurate account.

Dews and Wenger (1977) showed that the effects of amphetamine on the rate of reinforced responding was approximated by a two parameter equation. The equation has the form

$$\log (d/bl) = a - b\log(bl), \tag{2}$$

where d is drug response rate, bl is baseline response rate, and a and b are fitted parameters. In words, Equation 2 says that the logarithm of the drug effect is a linear function with negative slope of the logarithm of the baseline response rate, where drug effect is defined as the ratio of drug and baseline response rates. For drugs that increase response rate, the negative slope implies an inverse relationship between drug effect and baseline response rate: relatively larger increases at lower response rates, or increases at low response rates and no change or even small decreases at high response rates. The parameters of the rate dependency equation (a and b) have not been given interpretations. However, Gonzalez and Byrd (1977) found that the magnitude of the slope parameter (b) was usually between 0.5 and 1.0. This means that the drug effect included a decrease in the range of response rates. For example, as b approaches 1.0 the rate dependency equation implies that the drug condition response rates approached a constant value, equal to the intercept, a, regardless of reinforcement rate.

Results that are consistent with the rate dependency equation are also consistent with the matching law based descriptions. There are several correspondences. First, a decrease in R_e (increase in reinforcement efficacy) means that response rates increased and that the increases were an inverse function of baseline response rate. Second, a decrease in k means that the range of response rates decreased. For example, if k shrinks by one-half then the range of response rates shrinks by one-half. Third, the response rate changes that correspond to a decrease in R_e yield the linear relationship described by the rate dependency equation (Equation 2). This is shown in Fig. 3.16.

On the right side of Fig. 3.16, response rate is plotted as a function of reinforcement rate. For the data in the top panel, hypothetical results, there was a decrease in R_e (from 50 to 5 reinforcers per hour). In the bottom panel there was a decrease in k as well as R_e (k decreased from 100 to 50 responses per minute). On the left side, the same data are graphed in terms of the rate dependency equation. On the x-axis is the logarithm of the baseline response rate: log $(kR/(R + R_e))$, and on the y axis is the logarithm of the ratio of drug to baseline response rates: log $((k'R/(R + R'_e))/(kR/(R + R_e)))$. Consequently, if rate changes that correspond to a decrease in R_e are graphed in terms of the rate dependency equation, there is an approximately linear relationship with negative slope between the logarithm of the drug effect and the logarithm of the baseline response rate. In other words, an increase in reinforcement efficacy in variable-interval schedule experiments produces the results that have been designated "rate dependent." (A rate dependency graph of an increase in R_e was not included in Fig. 3.16. It would plot as an approximately linear function with a positive slope.)

Figure 3.16 shows that the same data set can be described about equally well by the rate dependency equation and the matching law equation (although there are small but systematic deviations from the rate dependent predictions at high response rates). The data, though, were hypothetical so that it would be of interest to determine which account provides the more accurate account of experimental results. The two equations each have two free parameters so that they can easily be compared in terms of how well they fit the data, and, as is noted below, there are situations in which the matching law and rate dependent equation predict qualitatively different outcomes.

The rate dependency equation was fit to the data by the method of least squares. Figure 3.17 shows the results for the subjects that provided the median fit for a given dose level. The rate dependency prediction of a negative slope held for doses between 0.25 and 1.0 mg/kg. But at 2.0 and 3.0 mg/kg, R_e increased. This means that response rates decreased as an inverse function of reinforcement rate. The median fit for the rate dependency equation was $r^2 = 0.58$. This is

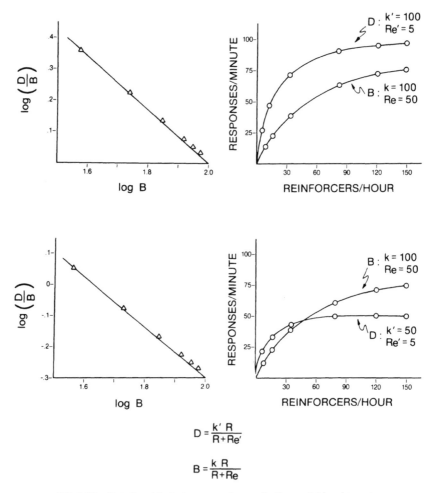

$$D = \frac{k' R}{R + Re'}$$

$$B = \frac{k R}{R + Re}$$

FIG. 3.16. Relationship between a change in the matching law parameter R_e and the rate dependency principle. The panels on the right
side show response rate as a function of reinforcement rate. In each
panel one curve shows baseline responding and the other curve
shows the response rates that correspond to a decrease in R_e (top
panel) and a decrease in R_c and k (bottom panel). In the left side panels,
the same results are graphed according the rate dependency principle.
There were small but systematic deviations from the predicted straight
line relationship at high baseline response rates.

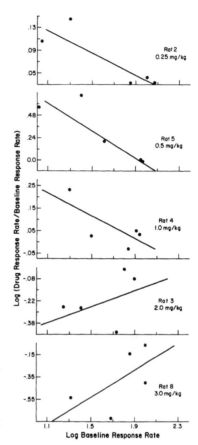

FIG. 3.17. A rate dependency description of the results from the amphetamine experiment. The panels show the subjects that provided the median fit at the indicated dose levels.

similar to what other researchers have obtained. We found four studies in which responding was maintained by variable-interval schedules and the rate dependency equation was used to describe the results (Beecher & Jackson, 1976; Bradshaw et al., 1981; Evans, 1971; Lucki, 1983). The median r^2 was 0.61. In contrast, the median fit for the matching law equation to this data set was $r^2 = 0.96$, and in 36 of 38 comparisons (5 drug levels, 8 subjects, and two instances in which subjects did not respond) the matching law equation description was more precise.

There are also situations in which the matching law equation and the rate dependency principle predict qualitatively different outcomes. For example, at high reinforcement rates, response rates typically approach an asymptotic level so that two very different reinforcement rates can be associated with virtually identical response rates. Under these conditions the rate dependency principle predicts similar changes since the response rates are nearly the same. However, the matching law approach says that identical baseline response rates can differentially change if they are associated with different reinforcement rates and there is a change in R_e. In a previous paper (Heyman & Seiden, 1986) this situation was examined, and it was found that nearly identical response rates differentially shifted when they were associated with different reinforcement rates.

ANTIDEPRESSANTS

In a review of animal models of depression, Willner (1984) concluded that procedures that use intra-cranial self-stimulation as the reinforcer were most promising. His assessment was, in part, based on the assumptions (1) that these procedures measured the reinforcing efficacy of brain stimulation, (2) that depression entails a loss of sensitivity to normally pleasurable activities, and (3) that there is a relationship between pleasure and reinforcement. These assumptions have support. First, the American Psychiatric Association's (1980) description of "major depressive episodes," begins with the sentence: "The essential feature is either a dysphoric mood, usually depression, or loss of interest or pleasure in all or almost all activities and pastimes." Second, there is evidence for a correlation between changes in the matching law measure of reinforcement efficacy and mood. Bradshaw and Szabadi (1978) obtained estimates of k and R_e from a manic depressive patient who participated in a variable-interval schedule experiment (five schedules per session, as we use). These estimates were compared to estimates of mood obtained from an 11-point rating scale. Increases in positive affect were correlated with decreases in R_e and increases in k.

Previous to our work there were two studies that used the matching law or a similar analysis to evaluate the effects of antidepressants on reinforced behavior. Fibiger and Phillips (1981) tested the effects of chronic desipramine treatment on responding maintained by brain stimulation reward. The subjects were rats and the procedure produced measures that are equivalent to k and R_e of the matching law. Chronic desipramine reduced the current level necessary for half-asymptotic responding (that is, it increased reinforcement efficacy). However, Jolly (1983, unpublished undergraduate thesis), using a procedure that was similar to the one used in the amphetamine and acute neuroleptic studies, found that desipramine increased R_e. The different outcomes may have been due to the deprivation conditions. Jolly's rats were water deprived and chronic desipramine appeared to make them sick: they ate less, lost weight, and one died. In contrast, Fibiger and Phillips' subjects were not deprived.

Using a procedure just like the one in the amphetamine and acute neuroleptic studies, we evaluated the effects of two atypical antidepressants: buproprion and nomifensine. Nomifensine was tested at doses from 0.375 to 5.0 mg/kg. Figure

NOMIFENSINE AND RESPONSE RATE

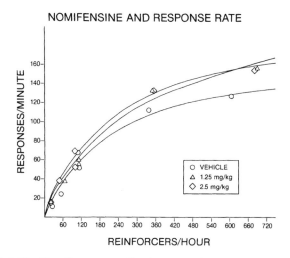

FIG. 3.18. The effects of nomifensine on reinforced responding. The open symbols show the group median response rates.

3.18 shows that the 1.25 and 2.5 mg/kg doses produced modest increases in response rate, and Fig. 3.19 shows that the increases were associated with an increase in motor performance factors. Doses below 1.25 had no discernible effects and doses above 2.5 led to inconsistent, sporadic responding. Buproprion was tested at doses of 5.0 to 40.0 mg/kg. However it produced no detectable change in either k or R_e.

There is evidence that nomifensine, buproprion, and desipramine increased reinforcement efficacy in studies in which the reinforcer was brain stimulation (e.g., Fibiger & Phillips, 1981; Gerhardt & Liebman, 1985; Liebman, Gerhardt, & Prowse, 1982). However in experiments in which behavior was maintained by water and the subjects were deprived, these drugs did not increase sensitivity to reinforcers. In contrast, neuroleptics and amphetamine affected reinforcement efficacy independently of the nature of the reinforcer and deprivation state. The sources for this difference are not known.

NEW DIRECTIONS: AVOIDANCE RESPONDING

De Villiers (1974) showed that the matching law predicted response rates in an avoidance procedure. In his study the subjects were rats, the shocks were presented according to a variable-interval timer, and a lever press eliminated the next programmed shock. Response rates were graphed as a function of the rate of shocks avoided, and the matching law equation approximated the relationship

NOMIFENSINE AND k AND Re

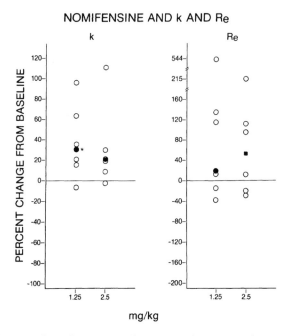

FIG. 3.19. The effect of nomifensine on the asymptotic response rates and rates of reinforcement that maintained a one-half asymptotic response rate (k and R_e). The filled symbols show the group medians. The asterik indicates a .05 significance level, according to the Wilcoxon test.

between these two variables (the mean r^2 was .98). We adapted this procedure in order to test the effects of drugs on avoidance responding.

Squirrel monkeys served as subjects. Each session consisted of five different variable-interval schedules, with each schedule in effect for 9 minutes. When an interval elapsed, a foot shock was delivered. However, if the monkey made a response, a lever press, the next scheduled shock was eliminated. That is, the interval simply elapsed so that responding reduced the frequency of shocks. The intervals varied from 120 sec (30 shocks per hour) to 2.5 sec (1440 shocks per hour). Nine minute time-out periods separated consecutive avoidance schedules. Figures 3.20, 3.21, and 3.22 show some representative results.

As with water and food deprived subjects, low doses of amphetamine increased responding, with response rates in the low reinforcement rate schedules showing relatively larger increases. This pattern of response rate change corresponds to a decrease in R_e. Thus amphetamine increased reinforcement efficacy for responding maintained either by the presentation of a positive reward or the removal of a negative reward.

The 1.5 mg/kg dose of chlorpromazine decreased response rates, with relatively larger decreases in the low reinforcement rate schedules, as in the water reinforcement study. This pattern of change corresponds to an increase in R_e. For example, for this subject the baseline parameter values were $k = 136$ responses/minute $(+/- 8)$ and $R_e = 997$ reinforcers/hour $(+/- 98)$, whereas at 1.50 mg/kg chlorpromazine the parameter values were $k = 179$ responses/minute $(+/- 26)$ and $R_e = 1863$ reinforcers/hour $(+/- 381)$, little less than a 100% increase.

Diazepam produced a different pattern of response rate changes than did either chlorpromazine or amphetamine. Response rates decreased proportionately. This is the pattern of response rate changes produced by increasing the weight of the lever, and it corresponds to a decrease in k. Thus, unlike amphet-

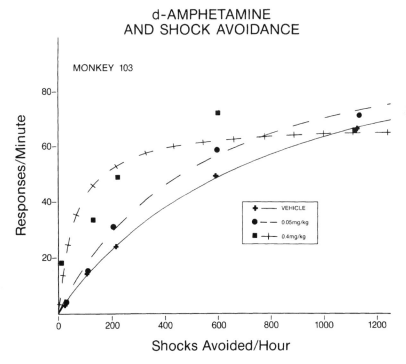

FIG. 3.20.   The effect of amphetamine on responding maintained by the avoidance of foot shock. The subject was a squirrel monkey and responses eliminated (avoided) a shock to the foot. The curves show the relationship between response rate and reinforcement rate (shocks avoided) predicted by the matching law equation.

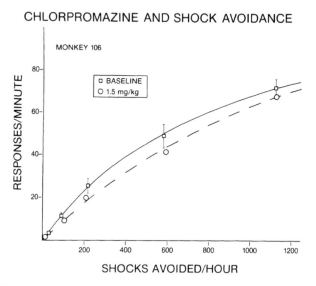

CHLORPROMAZINE AND SHOCK AVOIDANCE

SHOCKS AVOIDED/HOUR

FIG. 3.21. The effect of chlorpromazine on responding maintained by the avoidance of foot shock. The format is the same as in Fig. 3.20.

amine and chlorpromazine, diazepam reduced motor performance. This result may correspond to diazepam's clinical use as a muscle relaxant.

CAVEATS AND SUMMARY

Although methods based on the matching law equation have contributed to our understanding of the pharmacology of reinforced behavior, the approach has drawbacks. First, the experiments take a long time. In our laboratory, subjects have required about 40 to 60 sessions to obtain stable values of k and R_e. Moreover, k and R_e did not always remain strictly stable. In some subjects the parameters gradually drifted, and in others there were abrupt shifts to a new apparently stable level (Heyman & Monaghan, 1987; McSweeney, 1982). In 6 session samples, the average standard error for k was typically between 6 and 12% of its mean and for R_e the percentages were typically 16 to 22% (Heyman et al., 1986 and unpublished data). Second, matching law studies have invariably relied on an individual subject design. That is, each subject is exposed to each treatment level. This has advantages, but between-subject variability in sensitivity to the treatment can obscure an orderly dose-response curve. This may be corrected by normalizing the results, as in Fig. 3.15 or by using a group subject design. Group design studies have not been tried, but could prove helpful. Third, it may not be possible to obtain reasonable estimates of the matching law parameters if response rates at the two highest reinforcement rates do not approach an asymptote. Without an asymptote, the fitted curve may be more like a straight line than a hyperbola, and, as a result, the parameter estimates will be far outside the range of the observed response and reinforcement rates. Relatedly, it may not be possible to obtain reliable parameter estimates if there is a narrow range of response rates or if the relationship between response rate and reinforcement rate is non-monotonic. The general solution to the curve-fitting problems is is to use as small a serving of the reinforcer as possible and vary the rates of reinforcement over a wide range. This decreases the likelihood of large within session changes in satiation while increasing the likelihood of reinforcement rates that produce asymptotic response rates.

Although there are methodological problems, the matching law approach has been helpful. It was shown in this chapter that the matching law equation described the relationship between response rate and reinforcement rate independently of species, reinforcer, and deprivation state. For example, the equation

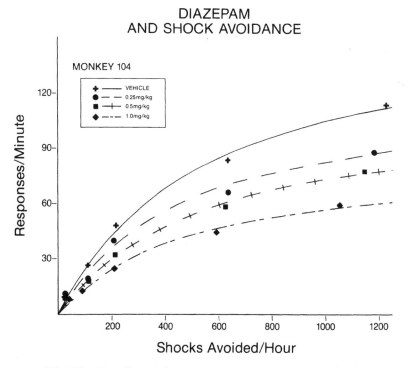

FIG. 3.22. The effect of diazepam on responding maintained by the avoidance of foot shock. The format is the same as in Fig. 3.20.

described the results from appetitive and avoidance procedures equally well, even though in one case a reinforcer is presented and in the other an aversive stimulus is removed. The behavioral pharmacology results were also quite general. Pimozide and chlorpromazine, which were the most widely tested neuroleptics, decreased reinforcement efficacy and slowed motor performance in studies that used different reinforcers, different deprivation conditions, and different response requirements. Amphetamine showed an equally broad generality, increasing reinforcement efficacy for food, water, brain stimulation, and shock avoidance. These findings make it sufficiently clear that certain neuroleptics and amphetamine alter an organism's capacity to be reinforced. This finding sets the stage, we believe, for several lines of research. The following projects seem to us most promising.

First, it would be informative to conduct studies in which the matching law method was combined with more precise biological manipulations. The results from these studies would provide biochemical and anatomical detail not available with systemic injections. Second, changes in reinforcement efficacy are open to further analysis. One path is suggested by the way many researchers have described operant behavior experiments. It is often assumed that an operant procedure is essentially a setting in which the subject chooses between the task the experimenter has arranged and other competing "background" activities, such as resting, exploring, preening, etc. (see, e.g., Baum & Rachlin, 1969: Herrnstein, 1970; McDowell, 1982). From this perspective, R_e is an index of the efficacy of the measured reinforcer relative to the background reinforcement (which is usually not directly measured). Evidence supports this formulation, for example, providing "extra" or free reinforcement increases R_e (Rachlin & Baum, 1972). Thus a drug induced change in R_e may entail a change in the efficacy of the measured reinforcer relative to the efficacy of competing reinforcers. For example, when amphetamine increased the efficacy of water reinforcement it may have done so by decreasing the reinforcing value of activities that competed with lever pressing, such as resting. This hypothesis has not been tested, nor its theoretical implications elaborated. Third, changes in the matching law parameters may have clinical significance. Bradshaw and Szabadi (1978) found that shifts in k and R_e were correlated with mood swings in a manic-depressive patient, and it is possible that the clinical effects of neuroleptics and stimulants are mediated by changes in reinforcement efficacy and/or motor performance. For example, attention is likely to depend, in part, on the reinforcing value of the impinging stimuli. Thus drugs that affect reinforcement processes may affect attentional processes, and, thereby, bring clinical relief.

In the introduction it was pointed out that experimental psychologists have developed techniques for identifying the behavioral mechanisms that mediate changes in reinforced behavior. In this chapter, we reviewed studies based on one of these analytical methods, the matching law equation. The results helped resolve one of the long-standing questions in behavioral pharmacology: whether or not neuroleptics attenuated reinforcement processes. It was shown that according to the matching law criteria, chlorpromazine pimozide, and fluphenazine decanoate attenuated both reinforcement efficacy and motor performance, but that low doses of cis-flupentixol acted on motor performance without reducing reinforcement efficacy. The matching law equation also led to a reinterpretation of one of the fundamental empirical findings in behavioral pharmacology. It was shown that a decrease in the matching law parameter R_e predicted the rate dependency relationship. That is, according to the matching law criteria, rate dependency reflects an increase in reinforcement efficacy. The results from these matching law studies have, in turn, opened the door to a host of new queries. For example, what biochemical mechanisms account for cis-flupentixol's unique behavioral profile, and would higher doses or a chronic dosing regime lead to changes in reinforcement efficacy? Thus, this chapter, we believe, has demonstrated that the matching law equation offers behavioral pharmacology a a useful analytical tool for interpreting the effects that drugs have on reinforced behavior.

ACKNOWLEDGMENT

The initial phases of this research was supported by Lew Seiden of the University of Chicago. More recently our efforts have been supported by Bernie Beer, chairman of the CNS Department at Lederle Laboratories. We thank both for their interest, encouragement, and, above all, good humor.

REFERENCES

American Psychiatric Association. (1980). *DSM III—Diagnostic and statistical manual of psychiatric disorders*. A.P.A. Washington.

Baldessarini, R. J. (1980). Drugs and the treatment of psychiatric disorders. In A. G. Gilman, L. S. Goodman, & A. Gilman (Eds.), *The pharmacological basis of therapeutics* (pp. 391–447). New York: Macmillan.

Baum, W. M., & Rachlin, H. A. (1969). Choice as time allocation. *Journal of the Experimental Analysis of Behavior, 12*, 861–874.

Beecher, G. D., & Jackson, D., S. (1976). Rate-dependent effect of amphetamine in rats: extension to between subject effect. *Psychopharmacologia, 46*, 307–309.

Berlyne, D. E., Koenig, I. D. V., Hirota, T. (1966). Novelty, arousal, and the reinforcement of diversive exploration in the rat. *Journal of Comparative and Physiological Psychology, 62*, 222–226.

Block, M. C., & Fisher, A. E. (1975). Cholinergic and dopaminergic blocking agents modulate water intake elicited by deprivation, hypovolemia, hypertonicity, and isoproterenol. *Physiology, Biochemistry, and Behavior, 3*, 251–262.

Bradshaw, C. M., Ruddle, H. V., & Szabadi, E. (1981). Relationship between response rate and reinforcement frequency in variable-interval schedules: III. The effects of d-amphetamine. *Journal of the Experimental Analysis of Behavior, 36*, 29–40.

Bradshaw, C. M., & Szabadi, E. (1978). Changes in operant behavior in a manic-depressive patient. *Behavior Therapy, 9*, 950–954.

Bradshaw, C. M., Szabadi, B., Bevan, P. (1978). Relationship between response rate and reinforcement frequency in variable-interval schedules: The effect of the concentration of sucrose
reinforcement. *Journal of the Experimental Analysis of Behavior, 29,* 447–452.

Bradshaw, C. M., Szabadi, E., Ruddle, H. V., & Pears, E. (1983). Herrnstein's equation: Effect of
deprivation level on performance in variable-interval schedule. *Behavior Analysis Letters, 3,* 93–
100.

Clark, A. J. (1933). The mode of action of drugs on cells. London: Edward Arnold.

Conrad, D. G., & Sidman, M. (1956). Sucrose concentration as reinforcement for lever pressing by
monkeys. *Psychological Reports, 2,* 381–384.

Cooper, J. R., Bloom, F. E., & Roth, R. H. (1986). The biochemical basis of neuropharmacology
(pp. 293–295). New York: Oxford University Press.

Creese, I. (1983). Receptor interactions of neuroleptics. In J. T. Coyle & S. J. Enna (Eds.),
Neuroleptics: Neurochemical behavioral, and clinical perspectives (pp. 183–222). New York:
Raven Press.

Davey, G., & Cleland, G. (1982). Topography of signal-centered behavior in the rat: Effect of
deprivation state and reinforcer type. *Journal of the Experimental Analysis of Behavior, 38,* 291–
304.

de Villiers, P. A. (1974). The law of effect and avoidance: A quantitative relationship between
response rate and shock frequency reduction. *Journal of the Experimental Analysis of Behavior,
21,* 223–235.

de Villiers, P. A., & Herrnstein, R. J. (1976). Toward a law response strength. *Psychological
Bulletin, 83,* 1121–1153.

Dews, P. B. (1958). Studies on behavior. IV. Stimulant actions of methamphetamine. *Journal of
Pharmacology and Experimental Therapeutics, 122,* 137–147.

Dews, P. B., & Wenger, G. R. (1977). Rate-Dependency of the behavioral effects of amphetamine.
In T. Thompson & P. B. Dews (Eds.), *Advances in behavioral pharmacology* (Vol. 1, pp. 167–
227). New York: Academic Press.

Ettenberg, A., Koob, G. G., & Bloom, F. E. (1981). Response artifact in the measurement of
neuroleptic-induced anhedonia. *Science, 209,* 357–359.

Evans, H. L. (1971). Behavioral effects of methamphetamine and d-methyltyrosine in the rat.
Journal of Pharmacology and Experimental Therapeutics, 176, 244–254.

Fibiger, H. C. (1978). Drugs and reinforcement mechanisms: A critical review of the catecholamine
theory. *Annual Review of Pharmacology and Toxicology, 18,* 37–56.

Fibiger, H. C., Carter, D. A., & Phillips, A. G. (1976). Decreased intracranial self-stimulation
after neuroleptics or 6-hydroxydopamine: Evidence for mediation by motor deficits rather than by
reduced reward. *Psychopharmacology, 47,* 21–27.

Fibiger, H., & Phillips, A. (1981). Increased intracranial self-stimulation in rats after long term
administration of desipramine. *Science, 214,* 683–685.

Fischman, M. W., & Schuster, C. R. (1979). The effects of chlorpromazine and pentobarbital on
behavior maintain by electric shock or point loss avoidance in humans. *Psychopharmacology, 66,*
3–11.

Fowler, S. G., Filewich, R. J., & Leberer, M. R. (1977). Drug effects upon force and duration of
response during fixed-ratio performance in rats. *Pharmacology, Biochemistry and Behavior, 6,*
421–426.

Fowler, S. G., Gramling, S. E., & Liao, R. M. (1986). Effects of pimozide on emitted force,
duration, and rate of operant responding at low and high levels of required force. *Pharmacology,
Biochemistry, and Behavior, 25,* 615–622.

Franklin, K. B. J. (1978). Catecholamines and self-stimulation: Reward and performance deficits
dissociated. *Pharmacology, Biochemistry, and Behavior, 9,* 813–820.

Gallistel, C. R., & Davis, A. J. (1983). Affinity for the dopamine D2 receptor predicts neuroleptic potency in blocking the reinforcing effect of MFB stimulation. *Pharmacology, Biochemistry, and Behavior, 19,* 867–872.

Gallistel, C. R., & Karras, D. (1984). Pimozide and amphetamine have opposing effects on the reward summation function. *Pharmacology, Biochemistry, and Behavior, 20,* 73–74.

Gallistel, C. R., Shizgal, P., & Yeomans, J. S. (1981). A portrait of the substrate for self-stimulation. *Psychological Review, 88,* 228–273.

Gerhardt, S., & Liebman, J. M. (1985). Self-regulation of ICSS duration: Effects of anxiogenic substances, benzodiazepine antagonists and antidepressants. *Pharmacology, Biochemistry, and Behavior, 22,* 71–76.

Gonzalez, F. A., & Byrd, L. D. (1977). Mathematics underlying the rate-dependency hypothesis. *Science, 195,* 546–550.

Gramling, S. E., Fowler, S. C., & Collins, K. R. (1984). Some effects of pimozide on nondeprived rats licking sucrose solutions in an anhedonia paradigm. *Pharmacology, Biochemistry, and Behavior, 21,* 617–624.

Hamilton, A., Stellar, J. R., & Hart, E. B. (1985). Reward, performance, and response strength method in self-stimulating rats: Validation and neuroleptics. *Physiology and Behavior, 35,* 897–904.

Herrera-Marschitz, M., & Ungerstedt, U. (1984). Evidence that apomorphine and pergolide induce rotation in rats by different D1 and D2 receptor sites. *European Journal of Pharmacology, 98,* 165–176.

Herrnstein, R. J. (1970). On the law of effect. *Journal of the Experimental Analysis of Behavior, 13,* 243–266.

Herrnstein, R. J. (1974). Formal properties of the matching law. *Journal of the Experimental Analysis of Behavior, 21,* 159–164.

Herrnstein, R. J. (1979). Derivatives of matching. *Psychological Review, 86,* 486–495.

Heyman, G. M. (1983). A parametric evaluation of the hedonic and motoric effects of drugs: Pimozide and amphetamine. *Journal of the Experimental Analysis of Behavior, 40,* 113–122.

Heyman, G. M. (1988). How drugs affect cells and reinforcement affects behavior: Formal analogies. In R. Church, M. L. Commons, J. R. Stellar, & A. Wagner (Eds.), *Quantitative analyses of behavior: Vol. 7. Biological determinants of reinforcement and memory* (pp. 157–182). Hillsdale, NJ: Lawrence Erlbaum Associates.

Heyman, G. M., Kinzie, D. L., Seiden, L. S. (1986). Chlorpromazine and pimozide alter reinforcement efficacy and motor performance. *Psychopharmacology, 88,* 346–353.

Heyman, G. M., & Monaghan, M. M. (1987). Effects of changes in response requirement and deprivation on the parameters of the matching law equation: New data and review. *Journal of Experimental Psychology: Animal Behavior Processes, 13,* 384–394.

Heyman, G. M., Monaghan, M. M., & Clody, D. E. (1987). Low doses of cis-flupentixol attenuate motor performance in rats. *Psychopharmacology, 93,* 477–482.

Heyman, G. M., & Seiden, L. S. (1986). A parametric description of amphetamine's effect on response rate: Changes in reinforcement efficacy and motor performance. *Psychopharmacology, 85,* 154–161.

Hull, J. H. (1977). Instrumental response topographies of rats. *Animal Learning and Behavior, 5,* 207–212.

Hyttel, J., & Arnt, J. (1986). Characterization of dopamine and D1 and D2 receptors. In G. R. Breese & I. Creese (Eds.), Advances in experimental medicine and biology: Vol 204. *Neurobiology of central D1-dopamine receptors* (pp. 15–28). New York: Plenum.

Iversen, S. D., & Iversen, I. (1975). *Behavioral pharmacology.* New York: Oxford University Press.

James, W. (1890). *The principles of psychology.* New York: Holt, Reinhart, and Winston.

Jolly, D. (1983). *Matching law analysis of the antidepressant desipramine.* Unpublished undergraduate thesis, University of Chicago.

Kelleher, R. T., & Morse, W. H. (1968). Determinants of the specificity of behavioral effects of drugs. *Ergenbnisse der Physiologie, 60,* 1–56.

Liebman, J. M., Gerhardt, S., & Prowse, J. (1982). Differential effects of d-amphetamine, pipradrol and bupropion on shuttlebox self-stimulation. *Pharmacology, Biochemistry, and Behavior, 16,* 791–794.

Logan, F. A. (1960). *Incentive.* New Haven: Yale University Press.

Lucki, I. (1983). Rate-dependent effects of amphetamine on responding under random-interval schedules of reinforcement in the rat. *Pharmacology, Biochemistry, and Behavior, 18,* 195–201.

Lyon, M., & Robbins, T. W. (1975). The action of central nervous system drugs: A general theory concerning amphetamine effects. In W. Essman & L. Valzelli (Eds.), *Current developments in psychopharmacology* (pp. 79–163). New York: Spectrum.

McDowell, J. J. (1982). The importance of Herrnstein's mathematical statement of the law of effect in behavior therapy. *American Psychologist, 37,* 771–779.

McSweeney, F. K. (1978). Prediction of concurrent keypeck and treadle-press responding from simple schedule performance. *Animal Learning and Behavior, 6,* 444–450.

McSweeney, F. K. (1982). Predictions of concurrent schedule performance. *Behavior Analysis Letters, 2,* 11–20.

Morley, H. J., Bradshaw, C. M., & Szabadi, E. (1984). The effect of pimozide on variable-interval performance: A test of the 'anhedonia' hypothesis of the mode of action of neuroleptics. *Psychopharmacology, 84,* 531–536.

Parent, M., & Toussaint, C. (1983). Flupenxtixol versus haloperiodol in acute psychosis. *Pharmatherapeutica, 3,* 354–364.

Pickens, R. (1977). Behavioral pharmacology: A brief history. In T. Thompson & P. B. Dews (Eds.), *Advances in behavioral pharmacology: Vol. 1.* London: Academic Press.

Rachlin, H. C., & Baum, W. M. (1972). Effects of alternative reinforcement. Does the source matter? *Journal of the Experimental Analysis of Behavior, 18,* 231–241.

Robbins, T. W. (1981). Behavioural determinants of drug action: Rate dependency revisited. In S. J. Cooper (Ed.), *Theory in psychopharmacology, Vol. 1* (pp. 1–63). London: Academic press.

Scatchard, G. (1949). The attraction of proteins for molecules and ions. *Annals of the New York Academy of Science, 51,* 660–672.

Singh, A. N. (1984). Therapeutic efficacy of flupenthixol decanoate in schizoaffective disorder: A clinical evaluation. *Journal of International Medical Research, 12,* 17–22.

Snyderman, M. (1983). Bodyweight and response strength. *Behavior Analysis Letters, 3,* 255–265.

Stauning, J. A., Kirk, L., & Jorgensen, A. (1979). Comparison of serum levels after intramuscular injections of 2% and 1% cis (z)-flupentixol decanoate in Viscoleo. *Psychopharmacology, 65,* 69–72.

Swets, J. A., Tanner, W. P. Jr., & Birdsall, T. G. (1961). Decision processes in perception. *Psychological Review, 68,* 301–340.

Towell, A., Muscat, R., & Willner, P. (1987). Effects of pimozide on sucrose consumption and preference. *Psychopharmacology, 92,* 262–264.

Wilkinson, G. N. (1960). Statistical estimates in enzyme kinetics. *Biochemical Journal, 80,* 324–332.

Willner, P. (1984). The validity of animal models of depression. *Psychopharmacology, 83,* 1–16. 1–16.

Wise, R. A. (1982). Neuroleptics and operant behavior: The anhedonia hypothesis. *The Behavioral and Brain Sciences, 5,* 39–87.

Wise, R. A., Spindler, J., deWit, H., & Gerber, G. J. (1978). Neuroleptic-induced "anhedonia" in rats: Pimozide blocks reward quality of food. *Science, 201,* 262–264.

Wistedt, B., Jorgensen, A., & Wiles, D. (1982). A depot neuroleptic withdrawal study. Plasma concentration of fluphenazine and flupentixol and relapse frequency. *Psychopharmacology, 78,* 301–304.

Zis, A. P., & Fibiger, H. C. (1975). Neuroleptic-induced deficits in food and water regulations: Similarities to the lateral hypothalamic syndrome. *Psychopharmacology, 43,* 63–68.

Zarevics, P., & Setler, P. E. (1979). Simultaneous rate-independent and rate-dependent assessment of intracranial self-stimulation. Evidence for direct involvement of dopamine brain reinforcement mechanisms. *Brain Research, 169,* 499–512.

4 Behavioral Pharmacology of Compounds Affecting Muscarinic Cholinergic Receptors

Jeffrey M. Witkin*
NIDA Addiction Research Center

INTRODUCTION

Acetylcholine (ACh) is a neurotransmitter in various regions of the central nervous system (CNS), at ganglionic and postganglionic sites in the peripheral nervous system, and at the neuromuscular junction. In the periphery, transmission of ACh participates in the regulation of a host of autonomic functions, glandular and smooth muscle activity, as well as skeletal muscle contraction. In the central nervous system, the functions of ACh are not as clearly defined. At this level cholinergic neurons may serve in the control of movement, sleep, fluid intake, sexual behavior, reactions to stress, and other behaviors. The symptomatology of Huntington's and Alzheimer's disease appear to derive impetus from disruption of normal cholinergic function.

ACh receptors were historically the first neurotransmitter receptor to receive experimental and theoretical attention (Dale, 1914; Langley, 1878). Two types of ACh receptor have been identified by classical pharmacological and radioligand binding methods. Actions of ACh at nicotinic receptors are mimicked by nicotine. Pharmacological properties of ACh that are similar to those of the natural alkaloid muscarine are termed muscarinic and are triggered by the binding of ACh to muscarinic receptors.

Cholinergic receptors in the mammalian CNS are primarily muscarinic (Salvaterra & Foders, 1979). Behavioral effects of ACh, as shown in experiments in which the actions of ACh are prolonged by inhibiting its enzymatic hydrolysis by

---

*Address correspondance to: Preclinical Pharmacology, Addiction Research Center, P.O.Box 5180, Baltimore, MD 21224

cholinesterase inhibitors, appear to principally involve muscarinic receptors. In addition, muscarinic receptors underlie many of the effects of iontophoretically applied ACh (Krnjevic, 1974). Thus, although behavioral effects of drugs acting at nicotinic receptors can be quite profound (cf. Spealman & Goldberg, 1982; Spealman, Goldberg, & Gardner, 1981; Stitzer, Morrison, & Domino, 1970), it appears presently that muscarinic actions of ACh are more intimately involved in behavioral regulation. For example, loss of muscarinic receptors is thought to be one of the major contributors to some symptoms of Alzheimer's disease (Iversen, 1986; Johns et al., 1985).

Early ligand binding studies indicated that muscarinic receptors represented a homogeneous class of receptors (Hulme, Birdsall, Burgen, & Metha, 1978). In the past several years, binding studies with novel muscarinic antagonists have revealed a heterogeneous class of muscarinic binding sites (Birdsall & Hulme, 1983; Hammer & Giachetti, 1984). These have been termed M_1 and M_2 receptors (Goyal & Rattan, 1978) and have distinct localization in the periphery and in the CNS (Buckley & Burnstock, 1986; Caufield & Straughn, 1983; Cortes & Palacios, 1986; Spender, Horvath, & Traber, 1986).

Compounds affecting muscarinic cholinergic receptors can be classified into three categories based on their mechanism of action at the receptor: cholinesterase inhibitors, muscarinic agonists, and muscarinic antagonists (Taylor, 1985a, 1985b; Weiner, 1985). Cholinesterase inhibitors or anticholinesterase compounds inhibit the activity of various cholinesterases. Acetylcholinesterase catalyzes the hydrolysis of ACh to acetate and water and provides the major mechanism for the termination of the biological actions of ACh. Cholinesterase inhibitors thus prolong the actions of ACh at the receptor. As such this class of drugs may also have actions at nicotinic ACh receptors. Cholinesterase inhibitors belong to several chemical classes and inhibit enzyme activity in a reversible (e.g., physostigmine or eserine) or irreversible (diisopropylphosphofloridate or DFP) fashion. Muscarinic agonists mimick the actions ACh by binding directly to muscarinic receptors. Muscarinic agonists vary considerably in structure. Natural and synthetic compounds include muscarine, pilocarpine, arecoline, and oxotremorine in addition to ACh itself. Choline esters such as bethanechol and methacholine are also agonists at muscarinic receptors. Collectively, compounds whose actions resemble those of ACh are sometimes referred to as cholinomimetics. Muscarinic antagonists prevent actions of ACh by competing for binding sites of the muscarinic receptor. Compounds such as atropine, scopolamine, and benactyzine are representative antagonists and block the effects of muscarinic agonists.

The selectivity of compounds for muscarinic receptors ranges widely within each drug class. For example, whereas oxotremorine displays high muscarinic selectivity, other agonists such as carbachol have prominent nicotinic actions. Atropine, the prototype antimuscarinic, not only blocks the effects of ACh but also blocks effects induced by some noncholinergic stimuli (Krnjevic, 1974). In addition to their receptor specificity another important property of muscarinic compounds governing their behavioral activity rests upon their physical chemistry. Hydrophilic drugs generally penetrate the CNS only at relatively high concentrations. Hence peripheral muscarinic receptors can be substantially occupied at doses producing little CNS activity.

Muscarinic agents have several clinical uses. These include the treatment of disorders of the gastrointestinal tract, urinary bladder, respiratory tract, cardiovascular system, and eye. They are also used in cancer chemotherapy as antiemetics, in myathenia gravis, Parkinson's disease, motion sickness, and in the treatment of cholinergic poisoning (Taylor, 1985a, 1985b; Weiner, 1985). Drugs from a number of other pharmacological classes have prominent anticholinergic activity which may account for some of their pharmacology (e.g., tricyclic antidepressants).

Evidence from behavioral studies points to the possibility that cholinergic neurotransmission is involved in the control of some highly integrated behaviors. These include responses maintained by positive or negative reinforcement and behavior suppressed by punishment. Cholinergic processes may also guide the acquisition (learning) and retention (memory) of behavior (cf. Heise, 1987; Seiden & Dykstra, 1977). The distribution of ACh and the receptors upon which it acts are confined to discrete pathways in brain (Kellar et al., 1985; Woolf, Eckstein, & Butcher, 1984), indicating a potential physical basis for selectivity of behavioral control by the cholinergic nervous system.

Much of the evidence for cholinergic control of behavioral function comes from behavioral pharmacology. Through administration of pharmacologically specific cholinergic agents and the observation of their effects on precisely controlled behavior, behavioral pharmacologists are in a unique position to assess the involvement of cholinergic processes in the control of behavior. Combined with additional analytic techniques such as cellular recording, brain stimulation, and lesioning of CNS structures, behavioral pharmacology can ultimately provide the type of integrative analysis critical to these scientific objectives. The success of this endeavor to understand the regulation of responding by the cholinergic nervous system is dependent upon adequate investigations of the variables controlling behavior and the specificity of the compounds available for augmentation or reduction of cholinergic function. Although a range of basic drugs with good selectivity for the cholinergic system is available and the techniques required for a precise experimental analysis of behavior have been in place for some time, detailed investigation of the behavioral pharmacology of any particular behavior has, in general, not been made. It is relatively easy to observe the effects of a drug on a performance presumably requiring memory; a challenge is presented with the task of documenting the selectivity of drug action on memory, a specific behavioral action (see Carlton, 1984; Kelleher & Morse, 1968; Russell, 1969; Weiss & Heller, 1969; Witkin and Katz, 1989 for a discussion of behavioral specificity of drug action and analysis of mechanisms of behavioral effects of drugs). The present status of the behavioral pharmacology of cholinergic compounds is thus primarily descriptive. The foundation for more detailed inquiry is clearly available.

The present account summarizes recent experiments characterizing the behavioral pharmacology of muscarinic compounds. This summary concentrates specifically on behavior under the explicit control of schedules of reinforcement. In the first section, effects of cholinomimetics are described with a view toward analyzing central and peripheral nervous system components of action. The second part concentrates on several aspects of the behavioral pharmacology of muscarinic antagonists. The final sections describe some current work on compounds with specificity for muscarinic receptor subtypes.

Because this chapter is not intended to be a summary of all major work in these areas, the following additional sources may be referenced for a more thorough description: Bignami and Michatek (1978); Carlton (1963, 1969); De Feudis (1974), McMillan and Leander (1976); Pradhan and Dutta (1971); Russell, (1969); Seiden and Dykstra (1977); Spencer and Lal (1983); Weiss and Heller (1969).

CHOLINESTERASE INHIBITORS AND MUSCARINIC AGONISTS

There has been a fair amount of work on the behavioral pharmacology of enhanced muscarinic stimulation most of which has concentrated on cholinesterase inhibitors, as ACh itself does not readily enter the CNS upon systemic administration. In general, muscarinic agonists and cholinesterase inhibitors produce decreases in the rate of occurrence of schedule-controlled behavior which do not depend appreciably on the type of behavior under investigation. There are however a few reports of rate increases with these drugs and some suggestion that the schedule of reinforcement and event maintaining responding may determine qualitative differences in their effects (see McMillan & Leander, 1976; Olds & Domino, 1969b; Pradhan & Dutta, 1971; Seiden & Dykstra, 1977). Facilitation of some behaviors not under explicit schedule control, e.g., sexual behavior (Ahlenius & Larsson, 1985) and their promising effects in the attenuation of memory deficits in Alzheimer's disease and senile dementia of the Alzheimer type (Heise, 1987; Iversen, 1986; Johns et al., 1985) demonstrate the utility of cholinomimetics as pharmacological tools in behavioral pharmacology.

Centrally-acting muscarinic compounds typically also have prominent peripheral actions that could contribute to their behavioral effects. Much experimental attention has focused on localizing the action of these compounds to the central and/or peripheral nervous system. The availability of analogs that do not readily penetrate the blood-brain-barrier enable some refined experiments in this direction. The general approach to this problem has been two-fold. First, direct comparisons between the agonist and an analog, usually quaternary, which does not appreciably enter the CNS, are used to assess the behavioral effects of peripheral muscarinic stimulation in relation to both central and peripheral stimulation. Second, attempts to antagonize the behavioral effects of an agonist by muscarinic antagonists which possess different degrees of CNS penetration provide additional and corroborative information on this question. Where brain areas involved in behavior have been characterized direct application of compounds to these sites can also be of value.

From results of experiments along these lines, it has been concluded that the behavioral effects of muscarinic agonist and of cholinesterase inhibitors are due to their interaction with muscarinic receptors in the CNS (Domino & Olds, 1968; Janowsky et al., 1986; Pfeiffer & Jenney, 1957; Vaillant, 1964, 1967). For example, neostigmine is a quaternary analog of the cholinesterase inhibitor physostigmine that does not alter brain ACh levels or acetylcholinesterase activity at doses producing large changes in the periphery (Domino & Olds, 1968, Maayani, Egozi, Pinchasi, & Sokolovsky, 1978; Rosecrans & Domino, 1974). With few exceptions (cf. Wenger, 1979), physostigmine is more potent than neostigmine in decreasing responding under a number of schedules of reinforcement or decreases responding more than neostigmine at equivalent degrees of peripheral cholinesterase inhibition (Domino & Olds, 1968; Stark & Boyd, 1963). By itself, these results of experiments in rodents might suggest that whereas neostigmine produces its effects on behavior by its actions in the periphery, physostigmine does so principally through central mechanisms. However, this type of experiment cannot in and of itself rule out the possibility that part of the behavioral effects of physostigmine are of peripheral origin. Likewise, the observation that behavioral effects of physostigmine are unaltered by administration of the quaternary antimuscarinic, methylatropine, does not constitute definitive evidence that the CNS actions of the compound are responsible for its behavioral activity. Another possibility is that a given behavioral effect of muscarinic agonists or cholinesterase inhibitors is due to actions of the compound at both central and peripheral sites and that these actions function redundantly to affect performance. The following experiments illustrate these points.

Because cholinesterase inhibitors may exert their behavioral effects at muscarinic, nicotinic, or a host of noncholinergic sties (cf. Aprison, 1962; Carbera, Torrance, & Viveros, 1966; Goldberg, Johnson, & Knaak, 1965), experiments were conducted to directly compare behavioral effects of centrally- and peripherally-acting cholinesterase inhibitors with direct-acting muscarinic agonists with high specificity for muscarinic receptors in the CNS or in the periphery. Lever pressing of squirrel monkeys was maintained under a schedule of electric shock postponement (Witkin, 1989). Under the avoidance schedule, shock was never presented less than 20 sec after a response. Shock occurred ever 5 sec in the absence of responding and 20 sec after the last response. Figure 4.1 presents molar comparisons of effects of physostigmine and the quaternary analog, neo-

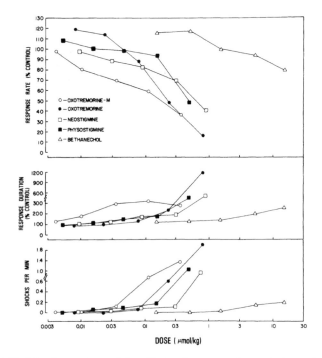

FIG. 4.1. Comparison of the effects of oxotremorine and physostigmine with their quaternary analogs oxotremorine-M and neostigmine
on avoidance responding of squirrel monkeys. Effects of the quaternary choline-ester, bethanechol, are also shown. Abscissa is molar
dose. Drug effects are means of single or duplicate determinations in 8
monkeys. From Witkin (1989) with permission.

stigmine on response rate, response duration, and rate of shock delivery. Effects
of the muscarinic agonist oxotremorine are shown in relation to a quaternary
analog, oxotremorine-M. Responding under the shock postponement-schedule
was decreased by all compounds; however, small response rate increases were
obtained in a few individual animals at the lower doses of oxotremorine or
physostigmine. These compounds also increased the duration of responses and
increased the rate of shock delivery. At higher doses, shocks were sometimes
presented repeatedly in the absence of responding. In addition, both the tertiary
and quaternary compounds produced pronounced peripheral parasympathetic
signs at the higher doses which included salivation, urination, diarrhea, and
emesis. Thus, both peripheral actions and behavioral effects were noted for the
tertiary compounds and their quaternary analogs with low CNS penetrability.
The only striking difference in the effects of the direct agonists with those of the
cholinesterase inhibitors was that the direct agonists produced behavioral effects

at doses somewhat lower than those inducing overt parasympathetic signs. Effects of bethanechol, a quaternary choline ester with high specificity for muscarinic receptors, were negligible; at the highest dose studied vomiting occurred.

On a molar basis physostigmine was equipotent with neostigmine in decreasing response rates by 50%; likewise oxotremorine and oxotremorine-M were equally potent in this regard (Fig. 4.1). Results of previous comparisons of behavioral effects of physostigmine and neostigmine have indicated that physostigmine has greater effects on behavior than neostigmine (Domino & Olds, 1968; Rosecrans & Domino, 1974; Stark & Boyd, 1963). On the other hand, Wenger (1979) found that neostigmine decreased food-maintained responding of mice at lower molar doses than physostigmine. Behavior of different species may thus be more or less sensitive to peripherally-acting anticholinesterase compounds. Any general statements regarding loci of cholinomimetic actions must be tempered with this caution.

Physostigmine was more potent than neostigmine in producing increases in shock rate or response duration. This is consistent with previous results indicating a greater behavioral effect of physostigmine than of neostigmine but contrasts with their equivalent potencies in decreasing response rate under the avoidance schedule. Thus, molar potency comparisons of behavioral effects of physostigmine and neostigmine depended upon the behavioral effect examined. The potency differences between physostigmine and neostigmine provide support for the independence of response rate, response duration, and shock rate as dependent measures of avoidance behavior and raise the possibility that distinct pharmacological properties of drugs may uniquely affect these measures. However, the pharmacological basis for the different sensitivities of the dependent measures to the effects of cholinomimetics is not clear. Whereas neostigmine was less potent than physostigmine in increasing shock rate, oxotremorine-M was more potent than oxotremorine in producing this effect. Thus, relative central or peripheral activation by these drugs did not reliably predict potency relationships.

Behavioral effects of bethanechol only occurred at a dose with pronounced peripheral parasympathetic actions (Fig. 4.1). This was unexpected since bethanechol, like oxotremorine-M, shows selectivity for peripheral muscarinic receptors, is relatively devoid of nicotinic effects and is only slowly degraded *in vivo* (Burleigh, 1978; Taylor, 1985a). The related compound, methacholine, and the quaternary cholinesterase inhibitor, pyridostigmine, also produce peripheral parasympathetic effects but minimal behavioral effects (Chalmers & Erikson, 1964; J. M. Witkin, unpublished observations). The lack of prominent behavioral effects of some quaternary cholinergic agents may be due to their selectivity at specific peripheral muscarinic receptors (Taylor, 1985a; Wess, Lambrecht, Moser, & Mutschler, 1984). Given the range of behavioral effects of quaternary compounds, definitive analysis of the contribution of CNS or peripheral mechanisms requires study of a series of related drugs.

All of the cholinomimetics studied had peripheral parasympathetic actions. The cholinesterase inhibitors produced their predominant behavioral effects in squirrel monkeys only at doses which produced concomitant peripheral effects. Only oxotremorine and oxotremorine-M produced behavioral effects at doses devoid of peripheral parasympathetic signs. Behavioral effects associated with peripheral signs were severe. At the highest doses, the monkeys often did not make any responses even in the presence of recurring shock. However, in squirrel monkeys responding under schedules of food presentation, physostigmine decreased responding at doses somewhat below those having severe overt parasympathetic activity (Chait & Balster, 1979; Witkin, Markowitz, & Barrett, 1989). Higher doses appear necessary to decrease avoidance responding. The intense behavioral demand of the avoidance baseline or the eliciting properties of shock may account for the difference in results with physostigmine under schedules of food presentation or electric shock postponement.

Effects produced by oxotremorine or physostigmine when given alone (open circles) or in conjunction (filled circles) with atropine, a muscarinic antagonist which acts in the CNS and in the periphery are shown in Fig. 4.2. Effects of drugs alone were essentially similar to those presented in Fig. 4.1. The * denotes the repeated occurrence of shock in the absence of responding (e.g., escape failure). Pretreatment with 1 mg/kg atropine prevented the response rate decreasing effects, as well as the increases in response duration and rate of shock delivery produced by oxotremorine and physostigmine. The effects of these drugs were prevented despite the fact that atropine had rate decreasing effects of its own (open squares). The increase in shock rate produced by physostigmine were not completely prevented by atropine. Parasympathetic signs were absent in atropine-treated monkeys. In addition, when atropine was given together with the higher doses of oxotremorine or physostigmine, response rates were increased substantially above control levels (see section on Muscarinic Antagonists–Behavioral excitatory effects, p. 101). The dose of oxotremorine studied in the presence of atropine was six-times higher than that studied alone. Despite the administration of sufficient atropine to completely prevent most behavioral effects and parasympathetic signs, four animals died unexpectedly 24 hours after the highest dose of oxotremorine (see Toxicity, p. 92).

Figure 4.3 shows the results of experiments with oxotremorine-M and neostigmine given alone (open circles) and in methylatropine-treated monkeys (filled circles). Oxotremorine-M and neostigmine also decreased responding under the avoidance baseline and increased response durations and the rate of shock presentation. As with oxotremorine and physostigmine, escape failures (*) were also seen at the higher doses. When given in the presence of 1 mg/kg methylatropine, a quaternary analog of atropine, effects of oxotremorine-M and neostigmine were prevented. This dose of methylatropine alone was without behavioral activity when given alone (open squares). Response rate increases after the combinations of these drugs with methylatropine were not significantly different

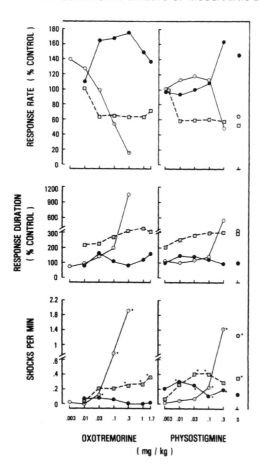

FIG. 4.2.   Effects of oxotremorine or physostigmine alone (○) or in combination with 1 mg/kg atropine (●) on avoidance responding of squirrel monkeys. Drugs were administered in cumulative doses at the beginning of each 10 min timeout period preceeding 10 min shock avoidance periods. Effects of 1 mg/kg atropine alone, given at the beginning of the first timeout period of the session, are indicated by the squares. Points above S represent effects of a saline injection given during the last timeout period; a cumulative dose of 0.3 mg/kg physostigmine had been given prior to the next to the last avoidance period. Recurrence of shock in the absence of responding is indicted by *. Drug effects are means of single or duplicate determinations in each of 5 (oxotremorine) or 8 (physostigmine) monkeys. From Witkin (1989) with permission.

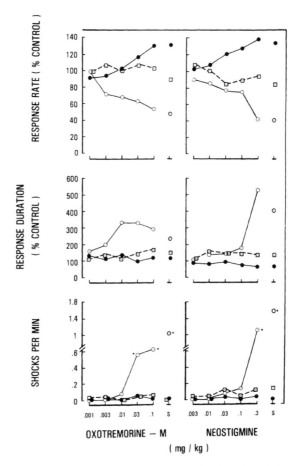

FIG. 4.3. Effects of oxotremorine-M or neostigmine alone (○) or in combination with 1 mg/kg methylatropine (●) on avoidance responding of squirrel monkeys. Effects of 1 mg/kg methylatropine alone, given at the begining of the first timeout period of the session, are indicated by the squares. Points above S represent effects of saline given during the last timeout period following the final cumulative dose of oxotremorine-M or neostigmine. Drug effects are means of single or duplicate determinations in each of 8 monkeys. Other details as in Fig. 4.2. From Witkin (1989) with permission.

than control. This contrasts with the more marked and significant response rate increases observed when atropine was combined with oxotremorine or physostigmine (Fig. 4.2). Peripheral signs produced by these compounds were not observed in methylatropine-treated monkeys.

Because 1 mg/kg methylatropine was an effective blocker of all peripheral parasympathetic effects of the quaternary cholinomimetics and of their behavioral effects, this dose of methylatropine was given in conjunction with oxotremorine and physostigmine in order to evaluate potential changes in the effects of these drugs when their peripheral muscarinic actions were sufficiently blocked. Figure 4.4 shows that the effects of neither oxotremorine nor physostigmine were modified by methylatropine.

Figure 4.5 presents representative cumulative response records illustrating that behavioral effects of the cholinomimetics were not only prevented by pretreatment with antimuscarinics but that they were also reversed by subsequent administration of muscarinic antagonists. Also seen in these records are the response rate increases with oxotremorine and physostigmine when given with atropine. The increases did not occur with oxotremorine-M or neostigmine given in conjunction with atropine.

Taken as a whole, these experiments indicate that the behavioral effects of physostigmine were primarily due to its muscarinic actions because the effects were blocked by atropine and were mimicked by direct-acting muscarinic agonists. In addition, the data suggest that the effect of physostigmine and oxotremorine on avoidance of squirrel monkeys were due to muscarinic activity in both the CNS and the PNS.

In the foregoing experiments, behavioral effects of oxotremorine or physostigmine resulting from their peripheral actions were studied by examining the effects of quaternary analogs. Had bethanechol been used as the only peripherally-acting muscarinic agonist, somewhat different conclusions regarding the mechanism of action of physostigmine and oxotremorine would have been required. The fact that the analogs oxotremorine-M and neostigmine were available made direct comparisons feasible. Effects of oxotremorine and physostigmine were, in all essential aspects, mimicked by neostigmine or oxotremorine-M. Effects of both neostigmine and oxotremorine-M were completely prevented by methylatropine. Prevention of peripheral actions of oxotremorine or physostigmine by methylatropine, however, did not alter the behavioral effects of these tertiary compounds despite the decreases in brain concentrations of oxotremorine which result from peripheral muscarinic blockade (Karlen, Traskman, & Sjoqvist, 1971). The absence of activity of methylatropine against oxotremorine or physostigmine stands in striking contrast to the complete prevention or antagonism of identical behavioral and peripheral parasympathetic actions of neostigmine or oxotremorine-M by methylatropine. Thus, whereas peripheral muscarinic activity of physostigmine and oxotremorine is an important component of their behavioral effects, peripheral actions are not necessary

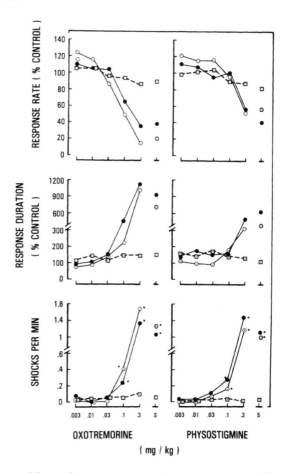

FIG. 4.4. Effects of oxotremorine or physostigmine alone (○) or in combination with methylatropine (●) on avoidance responding of squirrel monkeys. Points above S represent effect of saline given during the final timeout period of the session following the final cumulative dose of oxotremorine or physostigmine. Drug effects are means of single or duplicate determinations in each of 8 monkeys. Other details as in Fig. 4.3. From Witkin (1989) with permission.

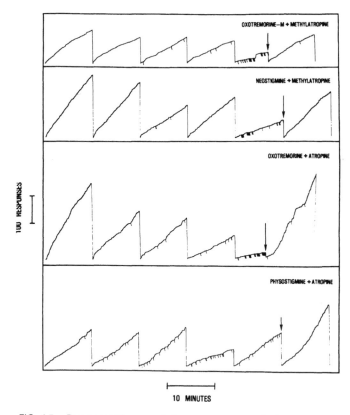

10 MINUTES

FIG. 4.5. Representative cumulative response records demonstrating the antagonism of the behavioral effects of oxotremorine-M or neostigmine by methylatropine (1 mg/kg) and antagonism of the behavioral effects of oxotremorine or physostigmine by atropine (1 mg/kg). Doses of muscarinic agonists or the cholinesterase inhibitors were given cumulatively at the beginning of each time-out period (doses are as depicted in Figs. 2 and 3). Atropine or methylatropine was administered 10 min prior to the avoidance period following the final cumulative dose of the test compounds (↓). The response pen incremented with each response and reset to baseline after either 400 responses or after the completion of each 10 min avoidance period. Responses during the 10 min timeout period separating each avoidance period were not recorded. Diagonal slashes on the records denote shock delivery. From Witkin (1987b).

for alterations in avoidance responding in squirrel monkeys. Central muscarinic actions of oxotremorine and physostigmine also contribute to their behavioral effects as evidenced by the prevention of their behavioral effects by the centrally-acting antimuscarinic atropine. Moreover, as adequate peripheral muscarinic blockade did not alter behavioral effects of physostigmine or oxotremorine, a simple additive model of central and peripheral muscarinic actions does not describe the behavioral effects of these drugs. Muscarinic receptors in the CNS and PNS appear to function redundantly in determining the behavioral effects observed in these experiments with squirrel monkeys.

The lack of prevention of the behavioral effects of physostigmine by quaternary antimuscarinics has been reported (Janowsky et al., 1986; Pfeiffer & Jenney, 1957; Vaillant, 1964, 1967). This observation has generally been interpreted as indicating that behavioral effects of physostigmine are centrally mediated. As already discussed, peripheral actions of physostigmine in and of themselves may also produce behavioral effects. The contribution of peripheral muscarinic actions to the behavioral effects of physostigmine was emphasized by the observations of Rosecrans, Drens, & Domino, (1968) and Rosecrans and Domino (1974) that methylatropine partially prevented the behavioral effects of physostigmine in rats.

Toxicity

Since the original report of Cho, Haslett, and Jenden (1962), there has been little evidence to suggest that oxotremorine has pharmacological actions in addition to its muscarinic agonist profile (Ringdaghl & Jenden, 1983). In squirrel monkeys death occurred unexpectedly after relatively high doses of oxotremorine when given in the presence of sufficient atropine to prevent the behavioral effects and peripheral symptoms of oxotremorine administration (Witkin, 1989). The dose of oxotremorine causing death was six times higher than that studied in the absence of atropine. Lethality was not likely the result of atropine. Atropine up to 10 mg/kg has been studied without any notable health effects in this species and a total of only 2 mg/kg was given in the experiment described earlier. This observation prompted investigation of the possible nonmuscarinic toxicity of oxotremorine (Witkin et al, 1987a).

With rats, oxotremorine in sufficient doses produces salivation, lacrimation, tremor, convulsions, and death. At 5 mg/kg oxotremorine and below, all of these effects were prevented by atropine. The tremor, convulsions and death occurring at higher doses of oxotremorine were not completely prevented or antagonized by antimuscarinics which readily blocked oxotremorine-induced salivation and lacrimation. The inability of atropine to prevent the toxicity of oxotremorine was not due to insufficient doses of atropine, time parameters, or routes of administration. Doses of atropine from 5 to 160 mg/kg i.p or 40 mg/kg s.c. were ineffective (Fig. 4.6). Lacrimation and salivation were completely prevented by

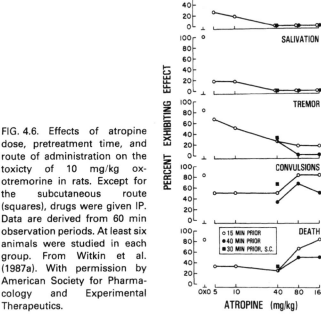

FIG. 4.6. Effects of atropine dose, pretreatment time, and route of administration on the toxicty of 10 mg/kg oxotremorine in rats. Except for the subcutaneous route (squares), drugs were given IP. Data are derived from 60 min observation periods. At least six animals were studied in each group. From Witkin et al. (1987a). With permission by American Society for Pharmacology and Experimental Therapeutics.

relatively low doses of atropine whereas, convulsions and death were not affected. In fact, higher doses of atropine were less effective blockers than lower doses.

In order to determine if the neurotoxicity of high oxotremorine doses was best characterized as atropine-insensitive or whether the convulsions and lethality were non-muscarinic in nature, three additional centrally-active muscarinic antagonists were evaluated. As with atropine, neither scopolamine, benztropine nor benactyzine were able to completely prevent neurotoxic effects of relatively high doses of oxotremorine even at dose levels sufficient to prevent peripheral parasympathetic actions (Fig. 4.7). For example, scopolamine was unable to completely suppress the convulsive activity of 10 mg/kg oxotremorine when given in doses sufficient to prevent salivation, lacrimation, tremor, and death. At higher doses of oxotremorine, tremor, convulsions and death occurred in a large percentage of animals despite administration of scopolamine in doses at least 16 times higher than required to completely prevent oxotremorine-induced lacrimation.

Benztropine and benactyzine produced the least protection against oxotremorine despite the greater central/peripheral antimuscarinic activity of these

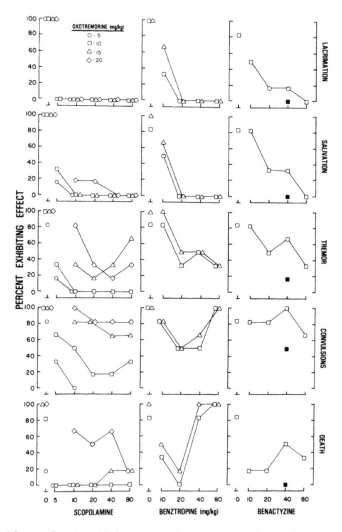

FIG. 4.7.   Relative abilities of scopolamine, benztropine, or benactyzine to prevent effects of different doses of oxotremorine (symbols defined in key). Data represent effects observed for 60 min after oxotremorine. Open symbols are effects obtained after a 15 min pretreatment with the antagonists; the solid squares show effects of a 40 min pretreatment for benactyzine. Effects of oxotremorine alone are shown as unconnected symbols above 0. At least six rats were studied in each group. From Witkin et al. (1987a). With permission by American Society for Pharmacology and Experimental Therapeutics.

compounds (Herz, Teschemachen, Hofstetter, & Kurz, 1965). With benac-tyzine, convulsions induced by 10 mg/kg oxotremorine were not significantly affected unless benactyzine was given 40 min prior to oxotremorine. Interesting-ly, methylatropine reduced lethality of oxotremorine without affecting tremor or convulsions (Witkin et al., 1987a). As with the tertiary antagonists, this differen-tial effect of methylatropine revealed that convulsions and lethality produced by oxotremorine are dissociable. The lethality of oxotremorine may thus be due at least in part to peripheral muscarinic receptors, perhaps those controlling car-diovascular parameters.

Results of experiments with two other muscarinic agonists, pilocarpine and arecoline, indicated that the nonmuscarinic neurotoxicity of oxotremorine was not unique to this compound (Witkin et al., 1987a). Thus, in high doses, struc-turally distinct muscarinic agonists have neurotoxic actions unresponsive to mus-carinic receptor blockade. It must be emphasized that whereas relatively high doses of these drugs have nonmuscarinic actions, effects of lower doses are blocked by muscarinic antagonists (Leander, 1981; Witkin, 1987a).

The possibility that actions of oxotremorine at nicotinic receptors were re-sponsible for the observed neurotoxicity, was discounted by the difference in the convulsive patterns between oxotremorine and *l*-nicotine and by absence of effect of the centrally-acting nicotinic antagonist, mecamylamine, against ox-otremorine-induced toxicity (Witkin et al., 1987a).

MUSCARINIC ANTAGONISTS

Numerous studies of the behavioral effects of antimuscarinics have been reported (see Bignami & Michatek, 1978; Carlton, 1969; McMillan & Leander, 1976; Seiden & Dykstra, 1977 for a summary of older data). In attempts to relate the antimuscarinic actions of antagonists *in vitro* with their behavioral effects, a series of compounds were compared in several assays (Witkin, Gordon, & Chian, 1987b). Figure 4.8 shows the structural formulas of the compounds studied. With the exception of methylatropine and pirenzepine, the compounds readily enter the CNS upon systemic administration. Both tropate (atropine and methylatropine) and benzilate (aprophen, adiphenine, benactyzine, ethylapro-phen, and azaprophen) antagonists were studied. Effects of selected compounds on responding under a fixed-ratio 10 schedule of food presentation in rats was determined.

Behavioral activity of the antimuscarinics is shown in Fig. 4.9. Dose-effect functions for azaprophen, aprophen, and benactyzine were steep and parallel. The muscarinic agonist oxotremorine displayed a similar slope to the dose-effect function but was more potent than any of the antagonists studied. Curves for the other compounds were flat across large portions of their dose range. With pi-

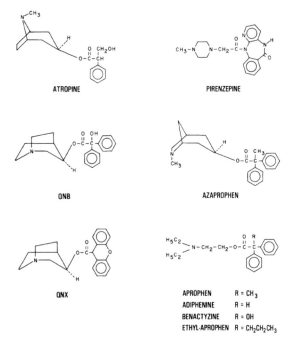

FIG. 4.8.   Structural formulas for the antimuscarinic agents studied. Methyl-atropine (not pictured) contains an additional methyl group on the nitrogen of atropine. From Witkin et al. (1987b). With permission by American Society for Pharmacology and Experimental Therapeutics.

renzepine, methylatropine, and adiphenine, decreases in response rates greater than 50% of control did not occur until relatively high doses.

In contrast to the other antimuscarinic agents studied, the benzilates, benactyzine, aprophen, and adiphenine, but not azaprophen, increased rates of responding (see also Boren & Navarro, 1959). The dose producing maximal increases in responding was about 10-fold lower than the ED_{50} for response rate decreases. Rate-increasing effects of these drugs were primarily the result of decreases in the period of no responding (pause) at the beginning of each fixed-ratio. The dose range of the compounds that did not increase rates (e.g., azaprophen) was extended to demonstrate that rate increases would not be observed at lower doses.

Similar rate-increasing effects of benzilate antagonists were observed in squirrel monkeys (G. Galbicka, R. A. Markowitz, J. E. Barrett, & J. M. Witkin, unpublished observations). Lever pressing was maintained under a multiple fixed-interval 3-min, fixed-interval 3-min schedule of food or electric shock delivery.

Under this schedule, the first response after 3 min produced food or a brief electric shock depending on whether red or white lights were illuminated. Although the temporal patterns of responding under the food or shock component were comparable, responding maintained by shock generally occurred at a higher rate than food-maintained responding under control conditions. Benactyzine, aprophen, and adiphenine increased rates of both food and shock-maintained responding (Fig. 4.10). Atropine and scopolamine produced dose-dependent decreases in responding under both conditions. The temporal pattern of responding under the fixed-interval schedules was disrupted by all compounds as evidenced by dose-dependent decreases in quarter-life values.

The potency relationships seen in Fig. 4.10 are similar to those observed in rats under a fixed-ratio schedule of food delivery (Fig. 4.9). The rate-increasing effects of adiphenine seen in both the squirrel monkeys and in rats suggests that previous conclusions regarding qualitative differences in the effects of adiphenine and benactyzine on schedule-controlled behavior may have been drawn without observation of an appropriate range of doses (Bignami, 1964; Boren, 1957). The increases in responding under both the food and shock schedules with the benzilates are comparable to the increases seen with psychomotor stimulants in squirrel monkeys under this baseline. In contrast, sedative-hypnotic drugs increase responding maintained by food but only decrease shock-maintained responding (see review by Barrett, 1985).

Although the data presented here point to a unique mode of action of the benzilate antimuscarinics (see also Fig. 4.7) which would have a structural as well as molecular basis (cf. Amitai et al., 1987), different conclusions may have

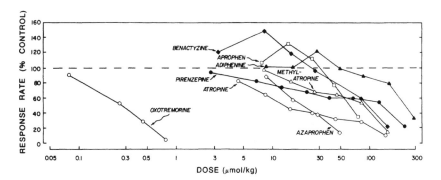

FIG. 4.9. Effects of selected muscarinic antagonists on responding of rats under a fixed-ratio 10 schedule of food delivery. Drug effects are shown in relationship to oxotremorine. Data are means of single or duplicate determinations in 6 or 8 animals (4 for azaprophen). From Witkin et al. (1987b). With permission by American Society for Pharmacology and Experimental Therapeutics.

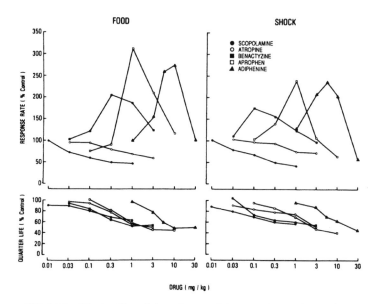

FIG. 4.10.   Effects of benzilate antimuscarinics, atropine, and scopolamine on responding of squirrel monkeys maintained under a multiple fixed-interval 3 min, fixed-interval 3 min schedule of food or electric shock presentation. Each point represents the mean effect of duplicate or triplicate determinations in two animals. From Galbicka, Markowitz, Barrett, and Witkin (unpublished).

been rendered had different behavioral performances been assessed. Galbicka and Witkin (unpublished observations) have observed that the presence of the schedule of shock presentation appears to make the increases in responding under the schedule of food delivery more likely. When studied in isolation, overall rates of responding under the fixed-interval schedule of food presentation were either unchanged or decreased by the benzilate compounds. However, under the multiple schedule of food and electric shock delivery, responding under the food schedule was substantially increased by the drugs as seen in Fig. 4.10.

Unlike the general durability of behavioral effects of cholinomimetics, antimuscarinic effects on behavior depend upon the conditions under which they are investigated. McKim (1973) showed that scopolamine increased responding under fixed-interval schedules of food presentation of rats and that the increases depended on the control rate of responding. Atropine and scopolamine are well known for their ability to increase low rates of responding in extinction where responding has no scheduled consequences (Carlton, 1963, 1969; Miczek, 1973; Russell, 1969; however, see McKim, 1980) and for their rate-increasing effects under some avoidance baselines (cf. Bignami & Michatek, 1978; McMillan &

Leander, 1976; Stone, 1964). Environmental or behavioral factors can also significantly alter the potency of drugs of this class. McMaster and Carney (1986) demonstrated that dose-effect functions for atropine and scopolamine under fixed-ratio schedules were shifted 10- to 40-fold to the right, respectively, in rats having 10 weeks of endurance exercise. The fact that scopolamine or atropine can increase responding under some conditions attests to the power of environmental and behavioral factors to modulate the behavioral activity of this class of drugs. This observation is consistent with the schedule-related determinants of the behavioral effects of drugs from a variety of pharmacological classes (Barrett & Katz, 1981; Kelleher & Morse, 1968; McMillan & Leander, 1976) and does not minimize the qualitative distinctions among these drugs previously discussed.

The qualitative difference in the effects of atropine and the benzilate antimuscarinics raised the possibility that their activity as antagonists of behavioral effects of agonist challenge may differ as well. In one experiment along these lines, lever pressing of rats was maintained under a fixed-ratio schedule of food presentation. Both atropine and aprophen functioned as antagonists of oxotremorine-induced behavioral inhibition (Witkin et al., 1987b). Atropine was 3-times more potent than aprophen in reversing the 92% response rate decrease produced by oxotremorine (0.79 μmol/kg); however, neither compound was able to alter the effects of this dose of oxotremorine by more than 64% (Fig. 4.11).

The intrinsic behavioral activity of the antagonists alone appeared to limit their activity as oxotremorine antagonists. The maximal efficacy of both compounds was reduced at doses which decreased responding when given alone.

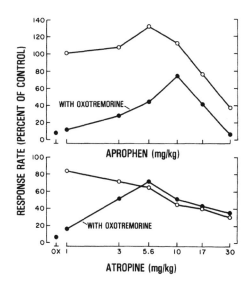

FIG. 4.11. Relative abilities of aprophen (top panel) or atropine (bottom panel) to reverse behavioral effects of 0.3 mg/kg oxotremorine (unconnected symbols above OX). Lever pressing of rats was maintained by food under a fixed-ratio 10 schedule. Open circles: aprophen or atropine alone; filled circles: antagonist effects when given 30 min prior to oxotremorine. Data are means of single or duplicate determinations in 6 or 8 animals. From Witkin et al. (1987b). With permission by American Society for Pharmacology and Experimental Therapeutics.

Response rate increases did not appear to markedly influence the activity of aprophen as an oxotremorine antagonist. Although 5.6 mg/kg aprophen maximally increased rates of responding, 10 mg/kg was required for maximal protection against oxotremorine. Dose-response functions for the behavioral effects of oxotremorine were shifted 3-fold to the right by either atropine or aprophen, although the area between the dose-effect curves was much greater for aprophen (Fig. 4.12).

Punished Responding

The increases in fixed-ratio responding seen with the benzilate antimuscarinics are also observed with sedative-hypnotic or anxiolytic agents (Wedeking, 1974; Witkin, 1984). With pentobarbital, increases of 20% were seen under the same conditions in which the antimuscarinics were studied (Witkin et al., 1987b). The possibility that benzilate antagonists would increase punished responding was therefore evaluated. Responding suppressed by punishment is increased by sedative-hypnotic and anxiolytic compounds (cf. Cook & Davidson, 1973; Kelleher & Morse, 1968; McMillan & Leander, 1976; Witkin, 1984) and benactyzine was reported to reported to have similar effects (Cook & Davidson, 1973). Lever pressing of rats was maintained under a multiple fixed-ratio 30 (food) fixed-ratio 10 (food + shock) schedule (cf. Witkin, 1984). Under this baseline, every 30th response in the presence of green lights produced food and every 10th response in the presence of red lights produced both food and shock. Responding was suppressed to about 90% of control levels by the punishment contingency. Nei-

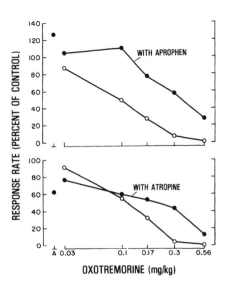

FIG. 4.12. Alteration in the behavioral effects of oxotremorine by aprophen (top panel) or atropine (bottom panel). Points above A represent effects of aprophen (10 mg/kg) or atropine (3 mg/kg) when given alone. Data are means of single or duplicate determinations in 6 or 8 animals. From Witkin et al (1987b). With permission by American Society for Pharmacology and Experimental Therapeutics.

ther atropine, aprophen, nor benactyzine increased punished responding (J. M. Witkin, unpublished observations) confirming the observation that muscarinic antagonists are generally devoid of this pharmacological property (cf. Bignami & Michatek, 1978; McMillan & Leander, 1976; Miczek, 1973).

Because a role for muscarinic receptors has been suggested for punished behavior from studies where antagonists were directly applied to the CNS (see Stein, Wise, & Belluzzi, 1977 for an overview), we investigated the possibility that systemically-administered muscarinic antagonists might potentiate the anti-punishment actions of the antianxiety compound chlordiazepoxide. In this study, 10 mg/kg atropine potentiated the rate-increasing effects of chlordiazepoxide (3 mg/kg) on punished responding. This dose of atropine decreased responding when given alone. Chlordiazepoxide blocked the rate-decreasing effects of atropine. Lower doses of atropine did not consistently potentiate the antipunishment effect of chlordiazepoxide. These data support previous observations implicating central muscarinic receptors in the control of behavior suppressed by punishment. The fact that central administration of atropine can increase punished responding suggests that the rate-decreases seen after systemic administration may be related to peripheral actions of the compound which are inconsistent with a sedative-hypnotic/anxiolytic profile. Aprophen did not alter the behavioral activity of chlordiazepoxide. This argues against a general role for muscarinic receptors in punished responding but is congruent with the different behavioral pharmacological profiles of these antagonists.

Behavioral Excitatory Effects

When physostigmine or oxotremorine were given in conjunction with atropine, rates of responding under a shock avoidance schedule were increased above control levels. Response rates were decreased when the drugs were given separately (Fig. 4.2). The response rate increases seen with oxotremorine or physostigmine in atropine-treated monkeys could have been the result of actions of either the cholinomimetics or of atropine that were unmasked by the other compound (Witkin, 1987). The response rate increases appear to be the result of actions of atropine which were revealed upon muscarinic receptor stimulation by either physostigmine or oxotremorine. For example, when studied under a multiple fixed-interval schedule of food or electric shock presentation, atropine decreases responding when administered immediately prior to experimental sessions as previously described (e.g., Fig. 4.10). However, when given at different times preceding sessions, atropine produces time-dependent increases in responding (Markowitz, Barrett, & Witkin, 1985; Witkin et al., 1989). Figure 4.13 shows that responding was increased to 200% of control values by atropine when given 2 hours prior to the experiment. The increases in rate and disruption of temporal patterning were not completely eliminated until a pretreatment time between 12 and 18 hours. The increases seen in Fig. 4.13 are of the same order

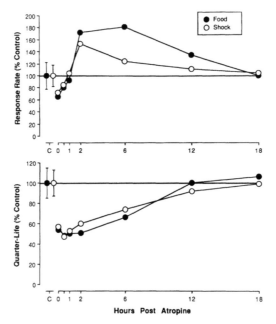

FIG. 4.13.   Effects of pretreatment time on behavioral effects of 1 mg/kg atropine. Responding of squirrel monkeys was maintained under a fixed-interval 3 min, fixed-interval 3 min schedule of food or electric shock presentation. Data are means of at least duplicate determinations in each of 4 monkeys. Vertical line represents ±1 S.D. Modified from Witkin et al. (1989) with permission.

of magnitude as observed when physostigmine or oxotremorine were combined with rate-decreasing doses of atropine (Fig. 4.2). Qualitatively similar time-dependent effects were also observed with scopolamine.

An initial evaluation of the involvement of muscarinic receptors in determining the rate-increasing effects of atropine was made by administering physostigmine in conjunction with atropine (Markowitz et al, 1985; Witkin et al., 1989). If both the rate-decreasing and rate-increasing effects of atropine are produced by similar mechanisms, physostigmine would be expected to alter the effects of atropine regardless of the time at which atropine is administered. The rate-decreases produced by immediate treatment with atropine were reversed by physostigmine (Fig. 4.14). In addition, under some dose combinations, response rates were increased above control levels. This effect was obtained even at doses of each compound that decreased responding when given alone. The temporal patterning (quarter-life) was not affected by physostigmine but remained depressed in atropine-treated monkeys when physostigmine was given. Although rate decreasing effects of atropine were reversed by physostigmine, increases in

response rates induced by appropriate pretreatment with atropine were not antagonized by physostigmine [unconnected symbols above 1.0 (2 hrs) in Fig.
4.14]. The decreases in quarter-life observed at 2 hour post atropine were likewise unaffected by physostigmine.

Response rate increases thus appear to be controlled by different mechanisms
than those related to the rate-decreasing effects of atropine. Whereas the rate
decreasing effects of atropine may involve muscarinic receptors, rate increases
may not. The enhancement of ACh turnover associated with atropine administration along with the observed increases in response rate seen under similar conditions with nicotine may be relevant to the behavioral excitatory effects of atropine. These presumed nicotinic actions would be revealed by appropriate
pretreatment times (allowing changes of ACh to be observed) or by administra-

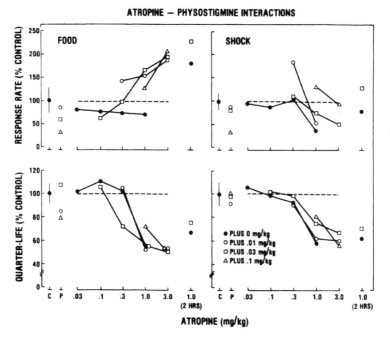

FIG. 4.14. Reversal of the rate-decreasing but not the rate-increasing
effects of atropine by physostigmine. Data are means of single or
duplicate determinations in each of four monkeys. Points above P
represent effects of physostigmine alone. Unconnected points above
1.0 (2 hrs) represent effects of 1 mg/kg atropine given 2 hr prior to
experimental sessions either alone or in combination with 0.03 mg/kg
physostigmine given at the begining of the session. All other drug data
are from injections given immediately prior to experimental sessions.
Other details as in Fig. 4.13. From Witkin et al. (1989) with permission.

tion of muscarinic agonists (blocking the rate decreases by competing for muscarinic receptors). Thus, nonmuscarinic behavioral excitatory actions of atropine may be expressed when the muscarinic-related decreases are blocked by either physostigmine or oxotremorine or when the decreases are overridden by excessive nonmuscarinic stimulation, perhaps triggered by time-dependent changes in ACh turnover. Since oxotremorine, with relatively few nicotinc actions, produces rate increases when given in conjunction with atropine, other noncholinergic actions may also be relevant to the observed behavioral excitation.

Whatever the mechanism, the increases in behavioral output seen after high doses of oxotremorine or physostigmine in the presence of atropine appear to be the result of central nervous system actions. Methylatropine, which had no effect alone, reversed all observed effects of neostigmine or oxotremorine-M without significantly increasing behavioral output above control levels (Fig. 4.3 and 4.5). Differences in the effects of combinations of muscarinic agonists and antagonists from the effects of either drug alone have been reported previously. Olds and Domino (1969a) reported that arecoline increased responding maintained by electrical brain stimulation when given in the presence of scopolamine. Increases in response rate after coadministration of drugs which do not themselves increase responding are not confined to cholinergic compounds. Meperidine decreased responding of squirrel monkeys when given alone but increased rate in the presence of naloxone or in morphine-tolerant animals (Witkin, Leander, & Dykstra, 1983). The rate increases seen with meperidine were thought to be due to proconvulsant actions which were revealed only after the rate-decreasing effects of meperidine were blocked by naloxone or morphine tolerance.

Additional variables have been identified which can modulate the behavioral effects of atropine. McKearney (1982) studied effects of drugs in squirrel monkeys responding under fixed-interval schedules of either food presentation or termination of a stimulus-shock complex. Atropine or scopolamine increased response rate to at least 150% of control in three or four of the ten monkeys studied. Biological factors or historical factors unrelated to genetics may therefore be a potential influence on the behavioral excitatory activity of this class of compounds. Galbicka and Witkin (unpublished observations) also have evidence to suggest that exposure to the rate-increasing effects of benzilate antimuscarinics may imbue atropine with large rate-increasing effects in squirrel monkeys.

It is unknown at present whether the rate-increases produced by benzilate antagonists share common mechanisms with those induced by atropine under the appropriate conditions. It is tempting, though realistically premature, to speculate that the behavioral excitatory effects of antimuscarinics may have some relationship to their psychotomimetic effects in man. Antimuscarinic drugs, especially benzilates like benactyzine, are well known for their CNS effects in man which include sedation, restlessness, excitement, delirium and hallucinations (Abood & Biel, 1962; Weiner, 1985). The propensity for some of these effects may be reflected in the behavioral excitatory effects observed in animal experiments.

Relation To In Vitro Actions

The relationship of the behavioral effects of the antimuscarinic compounds to some of their *in vitro* actions provided preliminary information on the role of muscarinic antagonist properties of these compounds as determinants of their behavioral effects. Behavioral activity was determined under a fixed-ratio 10 schedule of food presentation. ED_{50} values were derived from the dose-effect data presented in Fig. 4.9. The compounds were also evaluated for their ability to inhibit $[^3H]$N-methylscopolamine binding in N4TG1 neuroblastoma cells, ACh-induced contractions of isolated guinea-pig ilea, and carbachol-induced release of α-amylase from pancreatic acini (Witkin et al., 1987b). These data are summarized in Fig. 4.15. Only the relationship between α-amylase inhibition and behavioral effect was significant (center panel, r = 0.85; $p < 0.05$). However, if pirenzepine were excluded from the analysis, the correlation between inhibition of ileum contraction and behavioral effect was also significant (left panel, r = 0.80, $p < 0.05$). Pirenzepine was distinguished qualitatively from all other compounds in being more potent in its behavioral effects relative to its *in vitro*

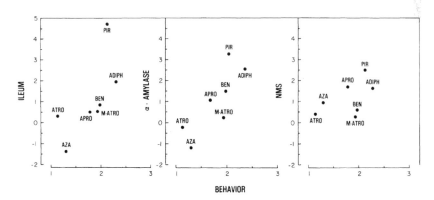

FIG. 4.15. Comparison of three *in vitro* properties with behavioral effects of selected antimuscarinic compounds. See text for details. Data are log potency values. Left panel: ileum vs. behavior; y = 2.86 x − 4.12; r = 0.667 ($p > 0.05$), Center Panel: α-amylase vs. behavior: y = 3.00x − 4.39; r = 0.848 ($p < 0.05$), N-methylscopolamine (NMS) binding vs. behavior: y = 0.89 x − 0.50; r = 0.517 ($p > 0.05$). M-ATRO: methyl atropine; ATRO: atropine; AZA: azaprophen; BEN: benactyzine; APRO: aprophen; ADIPH: adiphenine; PIR: pirenzepine. From Witkin et al. (1987b). With permission by American Society for Pharmacology and Experimental Therapeutics.

effects (the data for pirenzepine are to the left of a diagonal of slope 1.0). In the case of behavior vs. NMS binding, however, this difference was only ½ log unit (right panel, $r = 0.52$; $p > 0.05$).

Because the effects of the antagonists on fixed-ratio responding did not correlate precisely with their affinity for muscarinic receptors, we initiated some studies to examine more directly the role of muscarinic blockade to the behavioral effects of this class of drugs. The optical isomers, dexetimide and levetimide, were compared under a fixed-ratio 10 schedule of food presentation (K. Leach, G. Galbicka, & J. M. Witkin, unpublished observations). The levorotatory isomer is without appreciable affinity for muscarinic receptors. Dexatimide decreased response rates in a dose-dependent manner. A ¾ log difference in behavioral activity of the isomers was observed (Fig. 4.16). Levetimide produced very little effect until the highest dose, suggesting that its behavioral effects may not involve muscarinic receptors. Experiments are in progress to more fully characterize the differential effects of these and related drugs.

MUSCARINIC RECEPTOR SUBTYPES

Two subtypes of the muscarinic receptor are currently recognized, although uncertainty still exists regarding this classification (Nilvebrant, 1986). Cloning and sequence analysis of muscarinic receptor-encoding genes has uncovered four distinct gene products which may ultimately be determined to have the functional properties of muscarinic receptor subtypes (cf. Kerlavage, Fraser, & Venter, 1987). M_1 and M_2 subtypes appear to represent distinct proteins rather than unique conformations of the same receptor protein (Peralta et al., 1987). In the periphery, M_1 receptors are predominantly ganglionic, whereas postganlionic effector cells are primarily innervated with the M_2 subtype (Buckley & Burn-

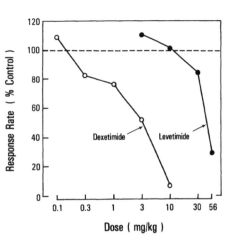

FIG. 4.16. Effects of dexetimide and the levorotatory isomer, levetimide, on responding of rats under a fixed-ratio 10 schedule of food presentation. Each point represents the mean of duplicate determinations in 5 rats. From Leach, Galbicka, and Witkin (unpublished observations).

stock, 1986; Caufield & Straughn, 1983). Brain localization of muscarinic receptor subtypes is also distinct. In rat brain, the highest density of M_1 receptors was detected in telencephalic structures, whereas M_2 receptors had a more diffuse central distribution (Spencer et al., 1986). Binding of muscarinic agonists produces a diversity of biochemical events including the inhibition of adenylate cyclase activity, phosphoinositide breakdown, and the regulation of K^+ and Ca^{+2} conductance (McKinney & Richelson, 1984). Neither the cellular events nor the postreceptor actions of muscarinic compounds are specifically linked to either receptor subtype in a consistent fashion across tissue types.

Pharmacological distinctions between M_1 and M_2 receptor subtypes may provide some additional insight into the manner in which actions of ACh at muscarinic receptors are translated into behavior. The discovery of subtypes of the muscarinic receptor also make possible the development of new compounds for precise physiological and behavioral endpoints. Pirenzepine, a selective antagonist at M_1 receptors, is a selective inhibitor of gastric acid secretion and is marketed in Europe as a novel anti-ulcer agent (Hammer & Giachetti, 1984; Hammer & Koss, 1979). Cardioselective activity is expressed by the M_2 antagonist AF-DX 116 (Micheletti, Montagna, & Giachetti, 1987). Muscarinic receptors are one of the primary receptors destroyed in Alzheimer's disease. Of the muscarinic receptors, the M_1 subtype is spared relative to the M_2 receptor in this disorder, making the development of cholinergic agonists with M_1 selectivity a reasonable drug-development goal (Iversen, 1986; Wess, Lambrecht, Moser, & Mutschler, 1987). Interestingly, pirenzepine, the prototypic M_1 antagonist, was 50 times more selective as an amnestic agent in mice (passive avoidance test) relative to its oxotremorine-antagonist properties; the nonselective antagonist, methylatropine, was not discriminating in its actions (Caufield, Higgins, & Straughn, 1983).

The ability of a series of muscarinic antagonists to inhibit [³H]N-methylscopolamine binding in N4TG1 neuroblastoma cells was compared to their potencies as antagonists of ACh-induced contractions of isolated guinea pig ilea (Witkin et al., 1987b). Figure 4.17 shows that pirenzepine and azaprophen did not display equivalent potencies across these assays as did most of the other compounds. Pirenzepine was relatively more potent as an inhibitor of [³H]N-methylscopolamine binding than as an inhibitor of ACh-induced ileum contractions; azaprophen had the opposite effects. In behavioral studies, pirenzepine was distinguished from other antimuscarinics in being relatively more potent in decreasing responding than in three *in vitro* assays (Fig. 4.15). Azaprophen again generally displayed the opposite relationship (Fig. 4.17). Since behavioral effects correlated with the potency of the antagonists to inhibit carbachol-elicited release of α-amylase from pancreatic acini (Fig. 4.15, middle panel) which display low affinity for pirenzepine (M_2), rate-decreasing activity of muscarinic antagonists may involve a similar or related set of muscarinic receptors. However, more refined studies are required to properly evaluate this idea.

FIG. 4.17. Comparison of inhibition of N-methylscopolamine (NMS) binding in N4TG1 neuroblastoma cells (log nM K_i) with inhibition of guinea-pig ileum contractions elicited by ACh (log nM k_B). Y = 0.95 x + 0.12; r = 0.726 (p < 0.05). The diagonal line indicates points of equivalence across measures (slope = 1.0). M-ATRO: methyl atropine; ATRO: atropine; AZA: azaprophen; BEN: benactyzine; APRO: aprophen; ADIPH: adiphenine; PIR: pirenzepine; E-APRO: ethyl-aprophen. From Witkin et al. (1987b). With permission by American Society for Pharmacology and Experimental Therapeutics.

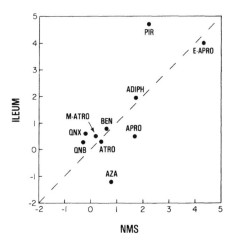

Azaprophen is a unique compound possessing both the benzilate structure of aprophen and the inverted tropane ring of atropine. It binds to the ACh anionic site in a manner not previously described for muscarinic antagonists and has exceptional antimuscarinic potency (Carroll et al., 1987). As previously described, azaprophen is also unique its *in vitro* actions and behavioral effects. Azaprophen may bind to a subset of muscarinic receptors distinct from those preferred by pirenzepine or interact in a unique fashion with an overlapping set of binding sites. The rate-increasing effects observed with aprophen are eliminated by replacement of the alkyl side chain of aprophen in azaprophen. Together with its high *in vitro* potency, its comparable potency to atropine in decreasing response rates, and the absence of response rate increases, it has been suggested that azaprophen may prove a useful antimuscarinic for clinic use with effective doses below those producing the side-effects of conventional antimuscarinics (Carroll et al., 1987; Witkin et al., 1987b).

Part of the deficit in our understanding of the functional relevance of muscarinic receptor subtypes at the integrated level of behavior rests in the lack of subtype-selective compounds which readily penetrate into the CNS upon systemic administration. Pirenzepine is a tricylic compound which differs in its physical chemistry from other centrally-acting tricyclic agents in being highly hydrophilic and hence penetrating into the CNS with difficulty (Hammer & Koss, 1979). Its limited CNS penetration by the systemic route may complicate the use of pirenzepine in behavioral pharmacology by requiring surgical technique to introduce the compound directly into brain (Caufield, 1983). Figure 4.18 compares dose-effect functions for the hydrophilic muscarinic antagonists

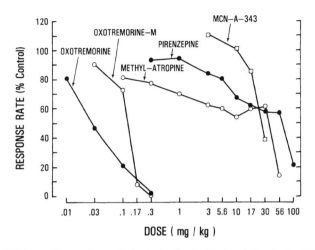

FIG.4.18. Comparison of the behavioral effects of the hydrophilic muscarinic antagonists, methylatropine and pirenzepine, in relation to the behavioral effects of three muscarinic agonists: oxotremorine, oxotremorine-M, and the quaternary M_1-selective agonist McN-A-343. Each point represents the mean effect of duplicate determinations in 6–12 rats responding under fixed-ratio 10 schedules of food delivery. All drugs were given IP either 30 min (methylatropine and pirenzepine) or immediately prior to experimental sessions. From Witkin et al. (1988). With permission of Pergamon Press.

pirenzepine and methylatropine in relation to those of three muscarinic agonists: oxotremorine, oxotremorine-M, and the M_1-selective agonist McN-A-343. Drug effects in rats were determined under a fixed-ratio 10 schedule of food presentation. Neither antagonist decreased responding beyond 50% of control except at high doses. McN-A-343 was devoid of striking behavioral effects except at 30 mg/kg where death occurred in 50% of the rats.

In order to evaluate potential central muscarinic antagonist properties of pirenzepine, its ability to prevent behavioral effects of oxotremorine or the peripherally-acting analog, oxotremorine-M, was determined. Methylatropine was compared to pirenzepine as an antagonist. Whereas methylatropine prevented behavioral effects of oxotremorine-M over a wide dose range, it was ineffective against the behavioral effects of oxotremorine confirming its peripheral muscarinic antagonist properties (Fig. 4.19). In contrast, pirenzepine prevented behavioral effects of both oxotremorine and oxotremorine-M (Fig. 4.20). Thus, pirenzepine may penetrate the CNS in sufficient concentrations to interact with central muscarinic receptors involved in the behavioral effects of oxotremorine. Systemically administered pirenzepine may be of potential utility as a tool for further investigation of the behavioral significance of M_1 receptors. For exam-

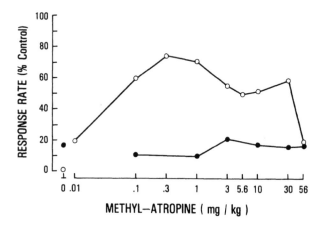

FIG. 4.19. Prevention of the behavioral effects of oxotremorine-M (○) but not oxotremorine (●) by methylatropine. Effects of oxotremorine-M or oxotremorine alone are shown as unconnected symbols above 0. Each point represents the mean effect of duplicate determinations in 6–12 rats. The dose of oxotremorine-M (1.09 μmol/kg) and oxotremorine (0.79 μmol/kg) was 0.3 mg/kg. At this dose, oxotremorine-M decreased responding to 1.1 ± 0.3 and oxotremorine to 17.2 ± 3.4% of control values. Injection details as in Fig. 4.18. From Witkin et al. (1988). With permission of Pergamon Press.

FIG. 4.20. Prevention of the behavioral effects of both oxotremorine-M (○) and oxotremorine (●) by pirenzepine. Effects of oxotremorine-M or oxotremorine alone are shown as unconnected symbols above 0. Oxotremorine-M decreased responding to 0.45 ± 0.12 and oxotremorine to 5.9 ± 1.1% of control values. Other details as in Fig. 4.19. From Witkin et al. (1988). With permission of Pergamon Press.

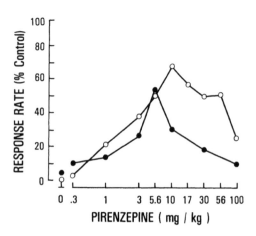

ple, the possibility of inducing selective memory impairments by M_1 receptor blockade without the need for elaborate behavioral preparations may facilitate progress on novel pharmacological treatments for Alzheimer's disease based upon the sparing of M_1 receptors (Iversen, 1986; Wess et al., 1987).

Some unique pharmacological properties of pirenzepine may also be responsible for its ability to antagonize the behavioral effects of oxotremorine. One possibility is the differential diffusion of these compounds to critical central structures. Methylatropine is preferentially taken up by cerebellum, pons, as well as preoptic and septal nuclei (Witter, Slangen, & Terpstra, 1973). Data on the regional uptake of pirenzepine into brain are not available; however, pirenzepine binds to an anatomical subset of binding sites in brain distinct from classic antimuscarinics (Cortes & Palacios, 1986). The M_1 receptor selectivity of pirenzepine may also be relevant to the observed antagonism of the behavioral effects of oxotremorine. Small concentrations of pirenzepine entering the CNS may, through selective interaction with central M_1 binding sites, account for the oxotremorine antagonism seen in Fig. 4.20.

It is important to note at this point that systemically administered methylatropine has been reported to antagonize carbachol-induced drinking in rats (Terpstra & Slangen, 1972). The antagonism of a centrally-mediated behavioral effect of carbachol is probably related to its high regional uptake into critical CNS areas. This observation underscores the fact that compounds which do not easily penetrate into brain may have prominent central actions. Caution must be exercised in interpreting drug effects based on limited pharmacological data. For example, given its diminished passage into the CNS alone, the observation that pirenzepine antagonizes behavioral effects of oxotremorine could have been interpreted as the antagonism of a behavioral effect of oxotremorine that was peripherally mediated. This conclusion is unlikely for several reasons. Pirenzepine was effective as an antagonist of oxotremorine-M across a wider range of doses than as an antagonist of oxotremorine. Methylatropine, in contrast to pirenzepine, was ineffective as an oxotremorine antagonist. Finally, the quaternary M_1 agonist McN-A-343 was behaviorally inactive up to toxic doses.

The possibility that the rate-decreases caused by McN-A-343 (30 mg/kg) represented a selective action upon M_1 receptors was cast further into doubt by the observation that pirenzepine did not alter either this behavioral effect or the lethality of McN-A-343 (Witkin et al., 1988). The lack of behavioral activity of McN-A-343 contrasts with the dose-related effects of other quaternary muscarinic agonists (e.g., neostigmine and oxotremorine-M) which are not subtype selective. Thus, M_1 sites in the periphery may be linked to select physiological (Wess et al., 1984) and behavioral functions.

Compounds available for study of M_2 receptors are also limited. The putative M_2 agonist AF-DX 116 was administered i.p. to rats responding under a fixed-ratio 10 schedule of food presentation. As with McN-A-343, AF-DX 116 had only minimal behavioral effects until a dose of 100 mg/kg. This dose decreased responding to 49% of control values without killing any of the rats.

The existence of multiple muscarinic receptor subtypes raises the potential for the development of highly selective ligands. Molecular biological approaches to this area of research have suggested the existence of four distinct subtypes. Transfection of tissue with a subtype-selective genome (cf. Peralta et al., 1987) may provide a unique tool for drug development. Given the flurry with which the pharmaceutical industry is encouraging progress in this area, as evidenced by their activity in the realm of autonomic drugs and compounds for Alzheimer's disease, the availability of experimental compounds of unique specificity is imminent. The next few years are likely to prove exciting in advancing our understanding of the behavioral significance of cholinergic neurotransmission. With this comes the promise of new therapeutic approaches to the management of behavioral dysfunction.

CONCLUSIONS

Behavioral effects of muscarinic compounds may not always be due to their interaction at muscarinic receptors. Some of the toxicology of agonists are also not adequately described in terms of their muscarinic receptor actions (Figs. 4.6 and 4.7). Despite considerable attention to the involvement of muscarinic receptors in the behavioral effects of cholinomimetics, little progress has been made on muscarinic antagonists. The lack of precise correlations of potencies *in vitro* with behavioral effects of antimuscarinic drugs raises the possibility that nonmuscarinic actions of the antagonist contribute to their behavioral effects (Fig. 4.15). Comparisons of behavioral potencies of optical isomers of muscarinic antagonists which differ in affinity for muscarinic receptors may help to clarify this problem (Fig. 4.16). However, only after detailed drug-interaction studies will closure be given to this question. The behavioral excitatory actions of antimuscarinics also do not appear to involve muscarinic receptors (Fig. 4.14). The generality and significance of this finding remains to be seen.

Definitive analysis of the involvement of muscarinic receptors or central vs. peripheral mechanisms in the behavioral effects of cholinergic drugs requires several pieces of information. Conclusions based on the results of individual experiments can be erroneous or misleading. For example, results of experiments comparing tertiary and quarternary cholinomimetics (Fig. 4.1) could have been interpreted as a peripheral mode of action for the behavioral effects of physostigmine or oxotremorine in squirrel monkeys. Likewise, the lack of antagonism of behavioral effects of these drugs by a peripherally-acting antimuscarinic (Fig. 4.4) has been interpreted in the opposite way; i.e., that peripheral muscarinic receptors do not participate in the observed effects of physostigmine or oxotremorine. However, the results of combined experimental approaches (Figs.

4.1–4.5) suggested a dual role of muscarinic receptors in the central and peripheral nervous systems in the behavioral effects of these drugs.

Behavioral effects of muscarinic antagonists are significantly influenced by the environmental conditions under which they are studied whereas the activity of cholinomimetics appear less malleable by behavioral factors. However, even for cholinomimetics, the type of behavior can determine the direction of behavioral change, potency relationships, and the relative importance of central and peripheral mechanisms.

Further analysis of the pharmacology of drugs selectively affecting muscarinic receptor subtypes may lead to new information on the cholinergic control of behavior and to the development of novel compounds targeted for precise physiological and behavioral endpoints.

Application of new methods in the experimental analysis of brain-behavior interactions will yield significant and novel insights into the relationship of cholinergic transmission and behavior. The implementation of these techniques and classical methods in the study of any precisely controlled behavior will, like the concentrated efforts of those tackling related problems (e.g., Kandel, 1985; Thompson, 1986), yield definitive answers to a puzzle with modern origins in the work of Langley, Dale, Eccles, Russell, Olds, Domino, Carlton, Heise, and others. Without dedicated and circumscribed efforts along these lines, however, our knowledge of these phenomena will not be expanded dramatically. Ironically, this is generally the way that we find ourselves presently, some 20 years after participants at a symposium sponsored by the American Society for Pharmacology and Experimental Therapeutics made similar pleas (cf. Russell, 1969; Weiss & Heller, 1969).

ACKNOWLEDGMENTS

I am grateful to R. Alvarado-Garcia, R. Crowley, and K. Leach for technical support and to G. Galbicka for his comments on an earlier draft of this paper. Discussion with J. E. Barrett, T. F. Elsmore, J. L. Katz, J. D. Leander, and K. M. Witkin were helpful in shaping some of the ideas presented in this manuscript.

REFERENCES

Abood, L. G., & Biel, J. H. (1962). Anticholinergic psychotomimetic agents. *International Review of Neurobiology, 4,* 218–273.

Ahlenius, S., & Larsson, K. (1985). Central muscarinic receptors and male sexual behavior: Facilitation by oxotremorine but not arecoline or pilocarpine in methscopolamine pretreated animals. *Psychopharmacology, 87,* 127–129.

Amitai, G., Herz, J. M., Bruckstein, R., & Luz-Chapman, S. (1987). The muscarinic antagonists aprophen and benactyzine are noncompetative inhibitors of the nicotinic acetylcholine receptor. *Molecular Pharmacology, 32*, 678–685.

Aprison, M. H. (1962). On the proposed theory for the mechanism of action of serotonin in brain. *Recent Advances Biological Psychiatry, 4*, 133–146.

Barrett, J. E. (1985). Behavioral pharmacology of the squirrel monkey. In L. A. Rosenblum & C. L. Coe (Eds.), *Handbook of squirrel monkey research* (pp. 315–348). New York: Plenum Press.

Barrett, J. E., & Katz, J. L. (1981). Drug effects on behavior maintained by different events. In T. Thompson, P. B. Dews, & W. A. McKim (Eds.), *Advances in Behavioral Pharmacology*, (Vol., 3 pp. 119–168). New York: Academic Press.

Bignami, G. (1964). Effects of benactyzine and adiphenine on instrumental avoidance conditioning. *Psychopharmacologia, 5*, 264–279.

Bignami, G., & Michatek, H. (1978). Cholinergic mechanisms and aversively motivated behaviors. In H. Anisman & G. Bignami (Eds.), *Psychopharmacology of aversively motivated behavior* (pp. 173–255). New York: Plenum Press.

Birdsall, N. J. M., & Hulme, E. C. (1983). Muscarinic receptor subclasses. *Trends in Pharmacological Sciences, 4*, 459–463.

Boren, J. J. (1957). Some effects of benactyzine upon operant behavior. *Journal of Pharmacology Experimental Therapeutics, 119*, 134–135.

Boren, J. J., & Navarro, A. P. (1959). The action of atropine, benactyzine, and scopolamine upon fixed-interval and fixed-ratio behavior. *Journal of the Experimental Analysis of Behavior, 2*, 107–115.

Buckley, N. J., & Burnstock, G. (1986). Autoradiographic localization of peripheral M1 muscarinic receptors using [^{3}H]pirenzepine. *Brain Research, 375*, 83–91.

Burleigh, D. E. (1978). Selectivity of bethanechol on muscarinic receptors. *Journal of Pharmacy and Pharmacology, 30*, 398–399.

Carbera, R., Torrance, R. W., & Viveros, H. (1966). The action of acetylcholine and other drugs upon the terminal parts of the postganglionic sympathetic fibre. *British Journal of Pharmacology and Chemotherapy, 27*, 51–63.

Carlton, P. L. (1963). Cholinergic mechanisms in the control of behavior by the brain. *Psychological Review, 70*, 19–39.

Carlton, P. L. (1969). Brain-acetylcholine and inhibition. In J. T. Tapp (Ed.), *Reinforcement and behavior* (pp. 237–286). New York: Academic Press.

Carlton, P. L. (1984). Analysis of physiological mechanism in psychopharmacology. *Neuropsychobiology, 12*, 158–172.

Carroll, F. I., Abraham, P., Parham, K., Griffith, R. C., Ahmad, A., Richard, M. M., Padilla, F. N., Witkin, J. M., & Chiang, P. K. (1987). 6-Methyl-6-azabicyclo[3.2.1]octane-3 α-ol 2,2-diphenylpropionate (azaprophen), a highly potent antimuscarinic agent. *Journal of Medicinal Chemistry, 30*, 805–809.

Caufield, M. P., Higgins, G. A., & Straughn, D. W. (1983). Central administration of the muscarinic receptor subtype-selective antagonist pirenzepine selectively impairs passive avoidance learning in the mouse. *Journal of Pharmacy and Pharmacology, 35*, 131–132.

Caufield, M., & Straughn, D. (1983). Muscarinic receptors revisited. *Trends in Neurosciences, 6*, 73–75.

Chait, L. D., & Balster, R. L. (1979). Effects of phencyclidine, atropine and physostigmine, alone and in combination, on variable-interval performance in the squirrel monkey. *Pharmacology Biochemistry and Behavior, 11*, 37–42.

Chalmers, R. K., & Erikson, C. K. (1964). Central cholinergic blockade of the conditioned avoidance response in rats. *Psychopharmacologia, 6*, 31–41.

Cho, A. K., Haslett, W. L., & Jenden, D. J. (1962). The peripheral actions of oxotremorine, a metabolite of tremorine. *Journal of Pharmacology and Experimental Therapeutics, 138*, 249–257.

Cook, L., & Davidson, A. B. (1973). Effects of behaviorally active drugs in a conflict-punishment procedure in rats. In S. Garattini, E. Mussini, & L. O. Randall (Eds.), *The benzodiazepines* (pp. 327–345). New York: Raven Press.

Cortes, R., & Palacios, J. M. (1986). Muscarinic cholinergic receptor subtypes in the rat brain. I. Quantitative autoradiographic studies. *Brain Research, 362,* 227–238.

Dale, H. H. (1914). The action of certain esters and ethers of choline and their relation to muscarine. *Journal of Pharmacology and Experimental Therapeutics, 6,* 147–190.

De Feudis, F. V. (1974). *Central cholinergic systems and behavior.* New York: Academic Press.

Domino, E. F., & Olds, M. E. (1968). Cholinergic inhibition of self-stimulation behavior. *Journal of Pharmacology and Experimental Therapeutics, 164,* 202–211.

Goldberg, M. E., Johnson, H. E., & Knaak, J. B. (1965). Inhibition of discrete avoidance behavior by three anticholinesterase agents. *Psychopharmacologia, 7,* 72–76.

Goyal, R. K., & Rattan, S. (1978). Neurohumoral, hormonal and drug receptors for the lower esophageal sphincter. *Gastroenterology, 74,* 598–618.

Hammer, R., & Giachetti, A. (1984). Selective muscarinic receptor antagonists. *Trends in Pharmacological Sciences, 5,* 18–20.

Hammer, R., & Koss, F. W. (1979). The pharmacokinetic profile of pirenzepine. *Scandanavian Journal of Gastroenterology, 14,* suppl. 57, 1–6.

Heise, G. A. (1987). Facilitation of memory and cognition by drugs. *Trends in Pharmacological Sciences, 8,* 65–68.

Herz, A., Teschemacher, H., Hofstetter, A., & Kurz, H. (1965). The importance of lipid-solubility for the central action of cholinolytic drugs. *International Journal of Neuropharmacology, 4,* 107–218.

Hulme, E. C., Birdsall, N. J. M., Burgen, A. S. V., & Metha, P. (1978). The binding of antagonists to brain muscarinic receptors. *Molecular Pharmacology, 14,* 737–750.

Iversen, L. L. (1986). The cholinergic hypothesis of dementia. *Trends in Pharmacological Sciences supplement, Subtypes of Muscarinic Receptors II:* pp. 44–45.

Janowsky, D. S., Risch, S. C., Kennedy, B., Zeigler, M., & Huey, L. (1986). Central muscarinic effects of physostigmine on mood, cardiovascular function, pituitary and adrenal neuroendocrine release. *Psychopharmacology, 89,* 150–154.

Johns, C. A., Haroutunan, V., Greenwald, B. S., Mohs, R. C., Davis, B. M., Kanof, P., Horvath, T. B., & Davis, K. L. (1985). Development of cholinergic drugs for the treatment of Alzheimer's disease. *Drug Development Research, 5,* 77–96.

Kandel, E. R. (1985). Cellular mechanisms of learning and the biological basis of individuality. In E. R. Kandel & J. H. Schwartz (Eds.), *Principles of neural science,* 2nd ed., (pp. 816–833). New York: Elsevier.

Karlen, B., Traskman, L., & Sjoqvist, F. (1971). Decreased distribution of oxotremorine to brain after pharmacological blockade of its peripheral acetylcholine-like effects. *Journal of Pharmacy and Pharmacology, 23,* 758–764.

Kellar, K. J., Martino, A. M., Hall, Jr., D. P., Schwatrz, R. D., & Taylor, R. L. (1985). High affinity binding of [^{3}H]acetylcholine to muscarinic cholinergic receptors. *Journal of Neuroscience, 5,* 1577–1582.

Kelleher, R. T., & Morse, W. H. (1968). Determinants of the specificity of behavioral effects of drugs. *Egerbnisse der Physiologie, Biologischen Chemie und Experimentallen Pharmakologie, 60,* 1–56.

Kerlavage, A. R., Fraser, C. M., & Venter, J. C. (1987). Muscarinic cholinergic receptor structure: Molecular biological support for subtypes. *Trends in Pharmacological Sciences, 8,* 426–431.

Krnjevic, K. (1974). Chemical nature of synaptic transmission in vertebrates. *Physiological Reviews, 54,* 418–540.

Langley, J. N. (1878). On the physiology of the salivary secretion. *Journal of Physiology* (Lond.), *1,* 339–369.

Leander, J. D. (1981).Antagonism of oxotremorine-induced behavioral suppression by anti-muscarinic drugs. *Psychopharmacology, 75,* 5–8.

Maayani, S., Egozi, Y., Pinchasi, I., & Sokolovsky, M. (1978). On the interaction of drugs with the cholinergic nervous system - V. Characterization of some effects induced by physostigmine in mice. *In vivo* and *in vitro* studies. *Biochemical Pharmacology, 27,* 203–211.

Markowitz, R. A., Barrett, J. E., & Witkin, J. M. (1985). Possible non-muscarinic behavioral effects of atropine in squirrel monkeys. *Federation Proceedings, 44,* 897.

McKearney, J. W. (1982). Effects of tricyclic antidepressant and anticholinergic drugs on fixed-interval responding in the squirrel monkey. *Journal of Pharmacology and Experimental Therapeutics, 222,* 215–219.

McKim, W. A. (1973). The effects of scopolamine on fixed-interval behaviour in the rat: A rate-dependency effect. *Psychopharmacologia, 32,* 255–264.

McKim, W. A. (1980). The effects of scopolamine on three different types of suppressed behavior of rats. *Pharmacology Biochemistry and Behavior, 12,* 409–412.

McKinney, M., & Richelson, E. (1984). The coupling of the neuronal muscarinic receptor to responses. *Annual Review of Pharmacology and Toxicology, 24,* 121–146.

McMaster, S. B., & Carney, J. M. (1986). Chronic exercise produces tolerance to muscarinic antagonist in rats. *Pharmacology Biochemistry and Behavior, 24,* 865–868.

McMillan, D. E., & Leander, J. D. (1976). Effects of drugs on schedule-controlled behavior. In S. D. Glick & J. Goldfarb (Eds.), *Behavioral pharmacology* (pp. 85–139). St. Louis: Mosby.

Micheletti, R., Montagna, E., & Giachetti, A. (1987). AF-DX 116, a cardioselective antagonist. *Journal of Pharmacology and Experimental Therapeutics, 241,* 628–634.

Miczek, K. A. (1973). Effects of scopolamine, amphetamine and chlordiazepoxide on punishment. *Psychopharmacology, 28,* 373–389.

Nilvebrant, L. (1986). On the muscarinic receptors in the urinary bladder and the putative sub-classification of muscarinic receptors. *Acta Pharmacologica et Toxicologica, 59,* suppl. 1, 1–45.

Olds, M. E., & Domino, E. F. (1969a). Comparison of muscarinic and nicotinic cholinergic ago-nists on self-stimulation behavior. *Journal of Pharmacology and Experimental Therapeutics, 166,* 189–204.

Olds, M. E., & Domino, E. F. (1969b). Differential effects of cholinergic agonists on self-stimula-tion and escape behavior. *Journal of Pharmacology and Experimental Therapeutics, 170,* 157–167.

Peralta, E. G., Winslow, J. W., Peterson, G. L., Smith, D. H., Henzel, W., Ashkenazi, A., Ramachandran, J., Schimerlik, M. I., & Capon, D. J. (1987). Primary structure and bio-chemical properties of an M_2 muscarinic receptor. *Science, 236,* 600–605.

Pfeiffer, C. C., & Jenney, E. H. (1957). The inhibition of the conditioned response and the counteraction of schizophrenia by muscarinic stimulation of the brain. *Annals of the New York Academy of Sciences, 66,* 653–764.

Pradhan, S. N., & Dutta, S. N. (1971). Central cholinergic mechanisms and behavior. *Internation-al Review of Neurobiology, 14,* 173–231.

Ringdahl, B., & Jenden, D. J. (1983). Pharmacological properties of oxotremorine and its analogs. *Life Sciences, 32,* 2401–2413.

Rosecrans, J. A., & Domino, E. F. (1974). Comparative effects of physostigmine and neostigmine on acquisition and performance of a conditioned avoidance behavior in the rat. *Pharmacology Biochemistry and Behavior, 2,* 67–72.

Rosecrans, J. A., Drens, A. T., & Domino, E. F. (1968). Effects of physostigmine on rat brain acetylcholinesterase and conditioned pole jumping. *International Journal of Neurophar-macology, 7,* 127–134.

Russell, R. W. (1969). Behavioral aspects of cholinergic transmission. *Federation Proceedings, 28,* 121–131.

Salvaterra, P. M., & Foders, R. M. (1979). $[^{125}I]_2$ α-Bungarotoxin and $[^3H]$ quinudiclinyl benzilate binding in central nervous systems of different species. *Journal of Neurochemistry, 32,* 1509–1517.

Seiden, L. S., & Dykstra, L. A. (1977). *Psychopharmacology: A biochemical and behavioral approach.* New York: Van Nostrand Reinhold.

Spealman, R. D., & Goldberg, S. R. (1982). Maintenance of schedule-controlled behavior by intravenous injections of nicotine in squirrel monkeys. *Journal of Pharmacology and Experimental Therapeutics, 223,* 402–408.

Spealman, R. D., Goldberg, S. R., & Gardner, M. L. (1981). Behavioral effects of nicotine: Schedule-controlled responding by squirrel monkeys. *Journal of Pharmacology and Experimental Therapeutics, 216,* 484–491.

Spencer, D. G., Jr., & Lal, H. (1983). Effects of anticholinergic drugs on learning and memory. *Drug Development Research, 3,* 489–502.

Spencer, D. G., Jr., Hovarth, E., & Traber, J. (1986). Direct autoradiographic determination of M1 and M2 muscarinic acetylcholine receptor distribution in the rat brain: Relation to cholinergic nuclei and projections. *Brain Research, 380,* 59–68.

Stark, P., & Boyd, E. S. (1963). Effects of cholinergic drugs on hypothalamic self-stimulation response rates in dogs. *American Journal of Physiology, 205,* 745–748.

Stein, L., Wise, C. D., Belluzzi, J. D. (1977). Neuropharmacology of reward and punishment. In L. L. Iversen, S. D. Iversen, & S. H. Snyder (Eds.), *Handbook of psychopharmacology,* vol. 8, (pp. 25–53). New York: Plenum Press.

Stitzer, M., Morrison, J., & Domino, E. F. (1970). Effects of nicotine on fixed-interval behavior and their modification by cholinergic antagonists. *Journal of Pharmacology and Experimental Therapeutics, 171,* 166–177.

Stone, G. C. (1964). Effects of drugs on non-discriminated avoidance behavior. *Psychopharmacologia, 6,* 245–255.

Taylor, P. (1985a). Cholinergic agonists. In A. G. Gilman, L. S. Goodman, T. W. Rall, & F. Murad (Eds.), *Goodman and Gilman's The pharmacological basis of therapeutics* (7th ed., pp. 110–129). New York: MacMillan.

Taylor, P. (1985b). Anticholinesterase agents. In A. G. Gilman, L. S. Goodman, T. W. Rall, & F. Murad (Eds.), *Goodman and Gilman's The pharmacological basis of therapeutics* (7th ed., pp. 110–129). New York: MacMillan.

Terpstra, G. K., & Slangen, J. L. (1972). The role of the tractus diagonalis in drinking induced by central chemical stimulation, water deprivation and salt injection. *Neuropharmacology, 11,* 807–817.

Thompson, R. F. (1986). The neurobiology of learning and memory. *Science, 233,* 941–947.

Vaillant, G. E. (1964). Antagonism between physostigmine and atropine on the behavior of the pigeon. *Naunyn-Schmiedeberg's Archives of Experimental Pathology and Pharmakology, 248,* 406–416.

Vaillant, G. E. (1967). A comparison of antagonists of physostigmine-induced suppression of behavior. *Journal of Pharmacology and Experimental Therapeutics, 157,* 636–648.

Wedeking, P. W. (1974). Schedule-dependent differences among anti-anxiety drugs. *Pharmacology Biochemistry and Behavior, 2,* 465–472.

Weiner, N. (1985). Atropine, scopolamine, and related antimuscarinic drugs. In A. G. Gilman, L. S. Goodman, T. W. Rall, & F. Murad (eds.), *Goodman and Gilman's The pharmacological basis of therapeutics* (7th ed., pp. 130–144). New York: MacMillan.

Weiss, B., & Heller, A. (1969). Methadological problems in evaluating the role of cholinergic mechanisms in behavior. *Federation Proceedings, 28,* 135–146.

Wenger, G. R. (1979). Effects of physostigmine, atropine and scopolamine on behavior maintained by a multiple schedule of food presentation in the mouse. *Journal of Pharmacology and Experimental Therapeutics, 209,* 137–143.

Wess, J., Lambrecht, G., Moser, U., & Mutschler, E. (1984). A comparison of the antimuscarinic effects of pirenzepine and N-methylatropine on ganglionic and vascular muscarinic receptors in the rat. *Life Sciences, 35,* 553–560.

Wess, J., Lambrecht, G., Moser, U., & Mutschler, E. (1987). Stimulation of ganglionic muscarinic M_1 receptors by a series of tertiary arecaidine and isoarecaidine esters in the pithed rat. *European Journal of Pharmacology, 134,* 61–67.

Witkin, J. M. (1984). Effects of some volatile sedative-hypnotics on punished behavior. *Psychopharmacology, 84,* 16–19.

Witkin, J. M. (1987). Non-muscarinic behavioral neurotoxicity of oxotremorine. In M. J. Dowdall & J. N. Hawthorne (Eds.), *Cellular and molecular basis of cholinergic function* (pp. 800–813). Chichester: Ellis Horwood Ltd..

Witkin, J. M. (1989). Central and peripheral muscarinic actions of physostigmine and oxotremorine on avoidance behavior of squirrel monkeys. *Psychopharmacology, 1989* (in press).

Witkin, J. M., Alvarado-Garcia, R., Lee, M. A., & Witkin, K. M. (1987a). Nonmuscarinic neurotoxicity of oxotremorine. *Journal of Pharmacology and Experimental Therapeutics, 241,* 34–41.

Witkin, J. M., Gordon, R. K., & Chiang, P. K. (1987b). Comparison of *in vitro* actions with behavioral effects of antimuscarinic agents. *Journal of Pharmacology and Experimental Therapeutics, 242,* 796–803.

Witkin, J. M., Alvarado-Garcia, R., Perez, L. A., & Witkin, K. M. (1988). Central oxotremorine antagonist properties of pirenzepine. *Life Sciences, 42:* 2467–2473, 1988.

Witkin, J. M., & Katz, J. L. (1989). Analysis of behavioral effects of drugs. *Drug Development Research* (in press).

Witkin, J. M., Leander, J. D., & Dykstra, L. A. (1983). Modification of behavioral effects of morphine, meperidine and normeperidine by naloxone and by morphine tolerance. *Journal of Pharmacology and Experimental Therapeutics, 225,* 275–283.

Witkin, J. M., Markowitz, R. A., & Barrett, J. E. (1989). Physostigmine-insensitive behavioral excitatory effects of atropine in squirrel monkeys. *Pharmacology Biochemistry and Behavior.*

Witter, A., Slangen, J. L., & Terpstra, G. K. (1973). Distribution of ^{3}H-methylatropine in rat brain. *Neuropharmacology, 12,* 835–841.

Woolf, N. J., Eckstein, F., & Butcher, L. L. (1984). Cholinergic systems in the rat brain I. Projections to the limbic telencephalon. *Brain Research Bulletin, 13,* 751–784.

5 Behavioral Responses Associated with Serotonin Receptors

Irwin Lucki
University of Pennsylvania

5-hydroxytryptamine (5-HT) has been implicated in the control of a wide array of both physiological and behavioral functions. 5-HT is involved in such diverse processes as pain perception, aggression, sleep, sexual behavior, hormone secretion, thermoregulation, cardiovascular function, motor activity, renal regulation, and food intake (for review, see Haber, Gabay, Issidorides, & Alivisatos, 1981; Jacobs & Gelperin, 1981; Osborne, 1982). 5-HT plays a key role in the pharmacological actions of antidepressant medications, antianxiety drugs, and hallucinogens. Given the widespread distribution of neurons containing this indoleamine in the central nervous system (CNS) (for review, see Azmitia, 1987), it is not surprising that 5-HT plays an important role in so many types of physiological functions.

The existence of multiple types of receptors may allow a single neurotransmitter like 5-HT to influence a wide range of behavioral functions by rendering more precise control over 5-HT's physiological effects. Multiple 5-HT receptors were described more than 30 years ago from studies of peripheral smooth muscle contraction (D and M receptors; Gaddum & Picarelli, 1957). More recently, radioligand binding techniques have made it possible to study CNS 5-HT receptors directly and have fueled an explosion of interest in 5-HT receptors and behavior. This chapter describes some of the more recent work indicating that 5-HT receptors classified using radioligand binding techniques are associated with specific behavioral responses. First, the current 5-HT receptor classification system and some of the most frequently-used selective compounds in recent behavioral experiments are described. Second, a large number of studies have employed behavioral responses elicited by injecting selective 5-HT agonists as models for the central activation of a selective receptor subtypes. Some of these studies, including some unpublished work from the author's laboratory, is discussed. Third, another group of studies employing the ability of animals to discriminate the stimulus properties of selective 5-HT agonists is reviewed. Finally, the implications of multiple 5-HT receptors for the study of 5-HT's role in naturally occuring behaviors are discussed.

MULTIPLE TYPES OF 5-HT RECEPTORS

Initial binding studies indicated the existence of two main classes of receptors for 5-HT: the 5-HT_1 receptor labeled by $^3\text{H-5-HT}$ and the 5-HT_2 receptor labeled by $^3\text{H-spiperone}$ or $^3\text{H-ketanserin}$ (Leysen, Niemegeers, Van Neuten, & Laduron, 1982; Peroutka & Snyder, 1979). Subsequent studies demonstrated that the 5-HT_1 receptor was not homogenous and at least four subtypes of this receptor have been identified, termed: 5-HT_{1A}, 5-HT_{1B}, 5-HT_{1C}, and 5-HT_{1D} (Heuring & Peroutka, 1987; Pazos, Hoyer, & Palacios, 1984; Pedigo, Yamamura, & Nelson, 1981). Newer methods employing selective ligands have been used to determine the affinity of a large number of 5-HT-related compounds for each receptor subtype (see Engel, Gothert, Hoyer, Schlicker, & Hillenbrand, 1986; Hall, El Mestikawy, Emerit, Pichat, Hamon, & Gozlan, 1985; Hoyer, Engel, & Kalkman, 1985a, 1985b; Leysen et al., 1982; Offord, Ordway, & Frazer, 1988; Peroutka, 1986; Sills, Wolfe, & Frazer, 1984). The D receptor of Gaddum and Picarelli (1957) was subsumed under the 5-HT_2 receptor and the M receptor may be associated with a third subtype called the 5-HT_3 receptor that is located principally in the periphery (Bradley et al., 1986).

One of the most useful recent compounds is 8-hydroxy-2-(di-n-propylamino) tetralin (8-OH-DPAT), a highly selective agonist at 5-HT_{1A} receptors without significant affinity for other 5-HT receptor subtypes or for most other neurotransmitter receptors (Engel et al., 1986; Middlemiss & Fozard, 1983; Neale et al., 1987). The piperidinyl indole agonist RU 24969 and the piperazine agonists 1-(m-trifluoromethylphenyl)piperazine (TFMPP) and m-chlorophenylpiperazine (m-CPP) are somewhat selective agonists at the 5-HT_{1B} receptor when their affinity is determined in the presence of guanine nucleotides (Sills et al., 1984) but TFMPP and m-CPP are also agonists at the 5-HT_{1C} receptor (Conn & Sanders-Bush, 1987). The phenylalkylamine compounds 2,5-dimethoxy-4-methylaphetamine (DOM), 2,5-dimethoxy-4-bromoamphetamine (DOB) and 2,5-dimethoxy-4-iodoamphetamine (DOI) were recently identified as agonists at both the 5-HT_2 receptor and the 5-HT_{1C} receptor (Titeler, Lyon, & Glennon, 1988). A number of 5-HT antagonists are available that are not selective between receptor subtypes, such as metergoline or methysergide. In contrast, ketanserin and ritanserin are relatively selective antagonists at 5-HT_2 receptors (Leysen et al., 1982). Mianserin and mesulergine are antagonists with high affinity for both the 5-HT_{1C} and 5-HT_2 receptor subtypes, whereas the beta-adrenergic antagonists pindolol and propranolol are selective for the 5-HT_{1A} and 5-HT_{1B} receptor subtypes (Engel et al., 1986; Nahorski & Willcocks, 1983).

The previous studies demonstrate that drugs show widely varying affinities for different 5-HT receptor subtypes. In addition, autoradiography studies have shown that these receptors are distributed differentially in brain (Marcinkiewicz et al., 1984; Pazos, Cortes, & Palacios, 1985). However, these binding studies fail to demonstrate directly that different 5-HT receptors mediate physiologically distinct functions. This role is reserved for functional studies. Consequently, the most recent studies of 5-HT-mediated biochemical (Conn & Sanders-Bush, 1987), neurophysiological (Sprouse & Aghajanian, 1987), and behavioral responses have focused on using drugs that binding methods reveal as being the most selective at 5-HT receptors in order to characterize distinct functional responses that are associated with 5-HT receptor subtypes.

The common goal of functional studies of 5-HT-mediated responses is to establish that agonist and antagonist potency relationships are related to their affinity for different 5-HT receptor subtypes. This objective for the pharmacologist studying behavior does not differ from that of pharmacological studies where the functional response involves biochemical or electrophysiological measures. However, this goal is not simply achieved because virtually none of the 5-HT agonists or antagonists presently identified can be considered specific or pure in their actions (see Fozard, 1987). Because the number of ideal 5-HT agonists or antagonists is limited, certain strategies can be outlined that enable important information to be obtained about behavioral responses and 5-HT receptor subtypes. (1) 5-HT-mediated behaviors can be studied using different agonists to establish potency relationships and to establish their common (or dissimilar) mechanism of action. (2) The effects of 5-HT antagonists with differing patterns of affinity for 5-HT receptors can be compared to establish the 5-HT receptor subtypes likely to mediate certain behavioral effects. For example, a comparison of the behavioral effects of two nonselective antagonists such as metergoline and methysergide with two selective 5-HT_2 antagonists such as ketanserin or pipamperone was originally used to establish that the 5-HT syndrome and head shaking behavior produced by 5-HT agonists in rats were mediated by 5-HT_1 and 5-HT_2 receptors, respectively (Lucki, Nobler, & Frazer, 1984). Subsequently, potency comparisons among several key antagonists, such as pindolol ($5\text{-HT}_{1A/1B}$), mianserin ($5\text{-HT}_{2/1C}$), and ketanserin (5-HT_2) may distinguish which 5-HT receptor subtypes mediate certain responses. (3) Comparisons of the effects of stereoisomers of agonists or antagonists can be used to determine whether their effects are associated with their affinity for 5-HT receptors.

UNCONDITIONED BEHAVIORS ELICITED BY 5-HT AGONISTS

Behavior changes in rodents elicited by the injection of 5-HT precursors or nonselective 5-HT agonists have been studied for nearly 30 years as whole-animal models for the stimulation of central 5-HT receptors. The recent availability of selective 5-HT agonists and antagonists has allowed some of these functional models to be identified with the activation of certain types of 5-HT receptors. Some of these studies are reviewed here.

5-HT Behavioral Syndrome

The administration to rats of drugs that enhance 5-HT neurotransmission produces a series of typical behavioral signs that are commonly called the 5-HT behavioral syndrome. The clearest definition of the 5-HT syndrome was proposed by Jacobs (1976) who defined the syndrome as the simultaneous display of 4–6 symptoms: (1) hindlimb abduction; (2) forepaw treading; (3) lateral head-weaving; (4) resting tremor; (5) hindlimb rigidity; and (6) Straub tail. If rats showed 4 of the 6 signs, they were rated as showing the syndrome in an all-or-none fashion. Additional behavioral signs of 5-HT receptor activation in rats have been studied by others, and included a typical low, outstretched posture, hyperreactivity, hyperactivity, intense salivation, backward walking, and pil-oerection. Our laboratory, and others (Sloviter, Drust, & Conner, 1978a) have used methods similar to those of Jacobs (1976), except that we rate the symptom of posture instead of limb rigidity to avoid handling the rats during study. The intensity of each symptom could also be rated individually (mild, moderate, or intense; 1–3) because individual symptoms may respond differently to pharmacological treatments (Dickinson, Jackson, & Curzon, 1983). In our laboratory, 4 out of the 6 symptoms must be present at moderate intensity (2) or greater to rate the animal as showing the 5-HT syndrome. Other laboratories focus ratings on the intensity of certain core symptoms such as forepaw treading, hindlimb abduction, or posture (see Deakin & Green, 1978; Tricklebank, Forler, & Fozard, 1985).

The 5-HT behavioral syndrome is caused by drugs that share the ability to activate 5-HT receptors (Jacobs, 1976). Administration of the 5-HT precursors tryptophan or 5-hydroxytryptophan (5-HTP) with a monoamine oxidase inhibitor (MAOI) cause the syndrome, but not if 5-HT synthesis is first prevented (Grahame-Smith, 1971). The 5-HT syndrome is also caused by drugs that enhance 5-HT release, such as fenfluramine or p-chloramphetamine (Trulson & Jacobs, 1976) and by 5-HT itself when injected into the intrathecal space of the spinal cord (Davis, Astrachan, & Kass, 1980). The dopamine agonists L-DOPA or amphetamine cause the syndrome at high doses, but appear to do so by enhancing the release of 5-HT (Deakin & Dashwood, 1981; Sloviter, Drust, & Conner, 1978b). The core symptoms of the 5-HT syndrome, except for headweaving, are associated with receptors located postsynaptically in the brain stem or spinal cord because: (1) the symptoms can still be produced following transections of the lower brain stem (Jacobs & Klemfuss, 1975); (2) the selective destruction of spinal 5-HT neurons enhances the ability of 5-HT agonists to cause the syndrome (Deakin & Green, 1978); and (3) local application of 5-HT into the intrathecal space of the spinal cord produces symptoms of the 5-HT syndrome (Davis et al, 1980).

Recent studies using selective agonists and antagonists have associated the 5-HT behavioral syndrome with the activation of the 5-HT$_{1A}$ receptor. Administration of the 5-HT$_{1A}$-selective agonist 8-OH-DPAT produces the 5-HT behavioral syndrome (Hjorth et al., 1982; Tricklebank et al., 1985). Ratings of the intensity for individual symptoms and the frequency of the syndrome following the injection of various doses of 8-OH-DPAT to rats in our laboratory are shown in Fig. 5.1. 8-OH-DPAT increased the intensity of each of the behavioral symptoms of the 5-HT syndrome and the percentage of animals demonstrating the syndrome in a dose-dependent manner. These effects are similar to behaviors caused by precursors of 5-HT synthesis or by other agonists such as 5-MeODMT or LSD (Lucki & Frazer, 1982a; Lucki et al., 1984).

Table 5.1 summarizes observations from our laboratory for the ability of 16 drugs that have been classified as 5-HT agonists to cause the 5-HT behavioral syndrome using a single strain of male Sprague-Dawley rats (Ace Animals; Boyertown, PA). In addition to the tetralin derivative 8-OH-DPAT, the 5-HT syndrome was produced by tryptamine derivatives, an ergot agonist (LSD),

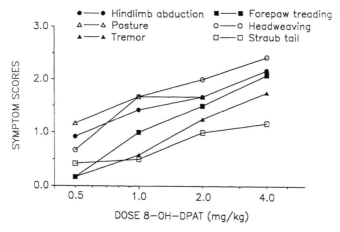

FIG. 5.1. Dose-effect curve for elicitation of the 5-HT behavioral syndrome following administration of various doses of the 5-HT$_{1A}$ agonist 8-OH-DPAT. The maximum intensity of each symptom was rated for a 15-min period following injection of 8-OH-DPAT according to the following scale: 3 = intense, 2 = moderate, 1 = mild, 0 = not at all. Rats were rated as showing the 5-HT syndrome at each dose of 8-OH-DPAT was: 0.5 mg/kg, 0%; 1.0, 25%; 2.0, 75%; and 4.0, 92%. Each point represents the mean symptom score or percentage frequency for different groups of 12 rats.

TABLE 5.1
Relative Ability of 5-HT Agonists to Produce the 5-HT Behavioral Syndrome[a]

Drugs That Cause the 5-HT Syndrome	ED50 Value (mg/kg)
d-lysergic acid diethylamide (LSD)	1.0
8-OH-DPAT	1.2
5-methoxy-3-(1,4,5,6-tetrahydrox-3-pyridyl)indole (RU 28253)	2.0
5-methoxy-N,N-dimethyltryptamine (5-MeODMT)	2.5
m-aminophenylethyl-TFMPP (m-APP)	6.7
p-aminophenylethyl-TFMPP (p-APP)	7.3
5-methoxy-3-(1,2,3,6-tetrahydro-4-pyridyl)-indole (RU 24969)	10.0
N,N-dimethyltryptamine (N,N-DMT)	15.0
N,N-diethyltryptamine (N,N-DET)	16.0

Drugs That Do Not Cause the 5-HT Syndrome	Highest Dose Examined (mg/kg)
Quipazine	10
6-chloro2-(1-piperazinyl)-pyrazine (MK 212)	10
1-(m-trifluroromethylphenyl)piperazine (TFMPP)	30
m-(chlorophenyl)piperazine (m-CPP)	30
2,5-dimethoxy-4-methylamphetamine (DOM)	8
2,5-dimethoxy-4-bromoamphetamine (DOB)	8
2,5-dimethoxy-4-iodoamphetamine (DOI)	8
Buspirone	20[b]
Ipsapirone	20[b]

[a]All drugs were adminstered by intraperitoneal injection to adult male Sprague-Dawley rats. Symptoms of the 5-HT syndrome were rated for the next 30 minutes and the occurrence of the syndrome was rated in an all-or-none manner as explained in the text. ED50 values are based on 4-point determinations of the dose-effect curve with each point consisting of 6–8 rats each.

[b]Only 2 symptoms, hind limb abduction and outstretched posture, were produced by buspirone and ipsapirone.

piperazine compounds, and the piperidinyl indoles RU 28253 and RU 24969 (Lucki, Sills, Frazer, & Nelson, 1987b). Among the compounds that did not cause the syndrome, injections of MK-212, m-CPP and TFMPP produce symptoms but only at lethal doses (Lucki & Frazer, 1982b; Lucki, Ward, & Frazer, 1989). Some of these observations differ from those performed by other laboratories. For example, quipazine has been reported to produce the 5-HT syndrome at doses of 25–50 mg/kg (Green, Hall, & Rees, 1981). However, these doses of quipazine were found to be toxic to rats in our laboratory and, in any event, confirm the lower potency of this drug to cause the 5-HT syndrome. The phenethylamine hallucinogens DOM and DOB were previously reported to produce the 5-HT syndrome (Sloviter, Drust, Damiano, & Conner, 1980), but we failed to observe symptoms up to doses (8.0 mg/kg) that greatly exceeded those required to produce head shaking behavior (0.1 mg/kg), a behavior mediated by 5-HT_2 receptors.

It is difficult presently to correlate the ability of 5-HT agonists to produce the 5-HT behavioral syndrome with their affinity for the 5-HT_{1A} receptor measured in binding studies. No laboratory has published data for all of the agonists using a single method and significant methodological differences exist between laboratories in binding procedures for the 5-HT_{1A} receptor (see Sills et al., 1984; Offord, DeAngelo, Wang, & Frazer, 1987). Furthermore, pharmacodynamic differences between agonists can produce different effects of drugs when they are injected systemically and compounds with high affinity for 5-HT_{1A} receptors may differ in their intrinsic efficacies once bound to the receptor. For example, the atypical anxiolytic drugs buspirone and ipsapirone have high affinity for the 5-HT_{1A} receptor but produce only the symptoms of hind limb abduction and body posture following systemic administration to rats (Lucki, 1986; Smith & Peroutka, 1986). Pretreatment with these drugs blocks production of the remaining symptoms of the 5-HT syndrome by 8-OH-DPAT (Lucki, 1986; Smith & Peroutka, 1986), suggesting that their partial agonist actions may sometimes block the effects of a full agonist such as 8-OH-DPAT. Nevertheless, it is interesting that the compounds in Table 1 that most potently caused the 5-HT behavioral syndrome possess relatively high affinity for the 5-HT_{1A} receptor (Asarch, Ransom, & Shih, 1985; Sills et al., 1984), whereas most of the agonists that did not cause the syndrome are less potent at the 5-HT_{1A} receptor (Sills et al., 1984; Titeler et al., 1988). These results suggest that affinity for the 5-HT_{1A} receptor is one factor that can influence whether directly-acting agonists produce the 5-HT behavioral syndrome.

Studies using 5-HT antagonists to block the 5-HT syndrome have also suggested involvement of the 5-HT_{1A} receptor. In one of the first studies to suggest a behavioral correlate for 5-HT_1 receptors, the 5-HT syndrome produced by 5-MeODMT was shown to be antagonized by nonselective 5-HT antagonists, such as metergoline or methysergide, but not by selective antagonists of 5-HT_2 receptors, such as ketanserin or pipamperone, even though the 5-HT_2 antagonists did block another 5-HT-related response, head shaking behavior (Lucki et al., 1984). Because the 5-HT_{1A} antagonist spiperone (Pedigo et al., 1981) was known to block the syndrome (Jacobs, 1974), the 5-HT_{1A} receptor was suggested to be associated with the 5-HT syndrome (Lucki et al., 1984).

Employing the 5-HT behavioral syndrome produced by 8-OH-DPAT (4.0 mg/kg) as a model for the activation of 5-HT_{1A} receptors, we recently examined the ability of a variety of 5-HT antagonists to block this behavioral effect. These data are shown in Fig. 5.2. As expected, the syndrome was potently blocked by the 5-HT_{1A} antagonist spiperone (ED50 = 1.8 mg/kg). The 5-HT syndrome was also blocked by ($-$)alprenolol (4.2 mg/kg), ($\pm$)pindolol (7.5 mg/kg), and ($\pm$)propranolol (18 mg/kg), in agreement with their high affinity for 5-HT_{1A}

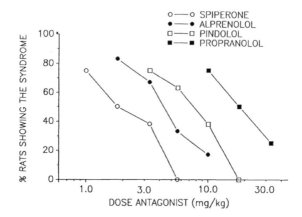

FIG. 5.2. Changes in body temperature produced by the administration of the 5-HT$_{1A}$ agonist 8-OH-DPAT to rats. Body temperature was measured by inserting a thermal probe 5 cm into the rectum. Rats were tested in individual cages and baseline values were determined following a 30-min habituation period. Each point represents the mean change in temperature from baseline values for a group of 6 rats at various times following the intraperitoneal administration of 8-OH-DPAT with vertical lines indicating 1 SEM.

receptors (Engel et al., 1986; Nahorski & Willcocks, 1983; Oksenberg & Peroutka, 1988). These results agree with a previous report that the 5-HT syndrome is antagonized selectively by the $(-)$ isomers of pindolol and propranolol (Tricklebank et al., 1985). Although these drugs are more potent antagonists of beta-adrenergic than 5-HT$_{1A}$ receptors, their order of potency to block the syndrome does not correlate with their affinity for beta-receptors (alprenolol = propranolol < pindolol; Tondo, Conway, & Brunswick, 1985). In contrast, pretreatment of rats with high doses (20 mg/kg) of the 5-HT$_2$ antagonists ketanserin, ritanserin, or mianserin failed to block elicitation of symptoms of the 5-HT syndrome by 8-OH-DPAT. This observation differs from that of Tricklebank et al. (1985) who reported that pretreatment with reserpine was necessary, for some reason, to prevent 5-HT$_2$ antagonists from blocking the 5-HT syndrome. Because our laboratory has never observed that 5-HT$_2$ antagonists block the 5-HT syndrome (Lucki et al., 1984; present report), we do not believe that pretreatment with reserpine is necessary to study the 5-HT syndrome when produced by the 5-HT$_{1A}$ agonist 8-OH-DPAT.

Temperature Regulation

In addition to stimulating postsynaptic 5-HT$_{1A}$ receptors, 8-OH-DPAT also activates presynaptic 5-HT$_{1A}$ autoreceptors located on the cell bodies of neurons containing 5-HT which would be expected to reduce the release of 5-HT from synaptic terminals. The ability of the 5-HT$_{1A}$ agonists 8-OH-DPAT, ipsapirone, and low doses of 5-MeODMT to produce marked reductions of body temperature in rodents have been used as a systemic assay for the activation of 5-HT$_{1A}$ receptors that are located presynaptically (Goodwin, De Souza, & Green, 1985a, 1986; Goodwin & Green, 1985; Gudelsky, Koenig, & Meltzer, 1986). Figure 5.3 illustrates the degree of hypothermia produced by 8-OH-DPAT given to rats. This hypothermic effect appears to be related to the activation of 5-HT$_{1A}$ receptors because a number of 5-HT$_{1A}$ antagonists, such as (−)pindolol, (−)propranolol, spiperone, or methiothepin prevent reductions of temperature by 8-OH-DPAT (Goodwin & Green, 1985; Gudelsky et al., 1986). The ICV administration of 8-OH-DPAT also reduces body temperature in mice and rats suggesting involvement of receptors located in the CNS (Goodwin et al., 1985a; Wieland, Goodale, & Lucki, submitted). The ability of 8-OH-DPAT to lower body temperature is thought to be due to its stimulation of 5-HT$_{1A}$ receptors located presynaptically because this effect is prevented by the inhibition of 5-HT synthesis with PCPA or by the destruction of 5-HT neurons (Goodwin et al., 1985a; Goodwin, De Souza, Green, & Heal, 1987). In contrast to the 5-HT behavioral syndrome, then, the hypothermic effect of 8-OH-DPAT appears to provide a functional indication of the stimulation of 5-HT$_{1A}$ presynaptic receptors. These actions of 8-OH-DPAT at presynaptic sites are important because they have been

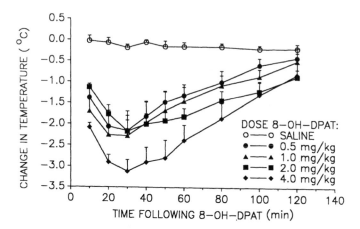

FIG. 5.3.   Blockade of the 5-HT syndrome by pretreatment with the 5-HT antagonists spiperone, (−)alprenolol, (±)pindolol, and (±)propranolol. The antagonists were administered 15 min prior to injection of the 5-HT$_{1A}$ agonist 8-OH-DPAT (4.0 mg/kg IP). Each point represents the value for a group of 8 rats. The method for rating the 5-HT syndrome was the same as described for Fig. 5.1. The 5-HT syndrome was produced by 4.0 mg/kg 8-OH-DPAT in 92% of rats tested without pretreatment (cf. Fig. 5.1).

suggested to mediate the effects of 5-HT$_{1A}$ agonists in preclinical screening tests for anxiolytic and antidepressant drug activity (Cervo & Samanin, 1987; Engel et al., 1984). However, other studies (Hjorth, 1985; Hutson, Donohoe, & Curzon, 1987) have failed to block 8-OH-DPAT's hypothermic effect in rats following severe depletion of 5-HT, so that the mechanism for 8-OH-DPAT reducing body temperature in rats is controversial.

Locomotor Activity

5-HT has long been thought to exert an inhibitory role in the control of locomotor activity in rodents because depletion of 5-HT content, by inhibiting 5-HT synthesis or by lesions of the raphe nuclei, causes dramatic increases in locomotor activity (see Gerson & Baldessarini, 1980). Although nonserotonergic elements may be involved in some of these effects (Lorens, 1978), the intraventricular injection of 5-HT reduces locomotor activity in rats (Green, Gillin, & Wyatt, 1976). Depletion of 5-HT potentiates the locomotor stimulatory effects of amphetamine (Lucki & Harvey, 1979) and central injection of 5-HT inhibits the effect of amphetamine (Warbritton, Stewart, & Baldessarini, 1978). However, the administration of 5-HT to rats or mice (pretreated with a peripheral decarboxylase inhibitor) stimulates locomotor activity (Modigh, 1972; Schlosberg & Harvey, 1979), and hyperlocomotion may accompany the production of the 5-HT syndrome (Grahame-Smith, 1971). Thus, manipulations of 5-HT on locomotor activity may differ depending upon the drug examined.

Administration of the 5-HT agonists, TFMPP, m-CPP, and MK 212 all produce reductions of the locomotor activity of unhabituated rats exposed to a novel environment (Lucki & Frazer, 1982b, 1985; Lucki et al., 1989). The activity suppression caused by TFMPP or m-CPP appears to be associated with the activation of 5-HT$_1$ receptors because pretreatment with nonselective antagonists, such as metergoline or methysergide, but not selective 5-HT$_2$ antagonists, such as ketanserin or pipamperone, block this behavioral effect (see Fig. 5.3; Lucki & Frazer, 1985). The behavioral effects of m-CPP and TFMPP can be distinguished from 5-HT$_{1A}$ agonists such as 5-MeODMT and 8-OH-DPAT because these piperazine agonists do not cause the 5-HT behavioral syndrome (see Table 5.1) and 8-OH-DPAT causes increases in locomotor activity (Lucki et al., 1989). Radioligand binding studies have shown that m-CPP, TFMPP, and MK 212 are more potent at the 5-HT$_{1B}$ and 5-HT$_{1C}$ receptors than 8-OH-DPAT (Conn & Sanders-Bush, 1987; Engel et al., 1986; Offord et al., 1988; Sills et al., 1984) and the selectivity of the piperazine agonists for these receptors may cause their different pattern of behavioral effects. Preferential involvement of the 5-HT$_{1C}$ receptor subtype is suggested by the ability of mianserin to block TFMPP's effects on locomotor activity (Fig. 5.4). In contrast, antagonists with high affinity for the 5-HT$_{1A}$ and 5-HT$_{1B}$ receptors, such as pindolol or propranolol,

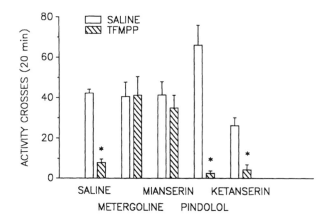

FIG. 5.4. The effect of pretreatment with different types of 5-HT antagonists on the ability of TFMPP to reduce locomotor activity in rats. Locomotor activity was measured for 20 min as the number of crosses along the longitudinal axis of an activity cage that was monitored by photocells connected to a microcomputer. Each vertical bar represents the mean number of crosses for groups of 6–8 rats, with vertical lines indicating 1 SEM. Open bars represent pretreatment with saline (0.9% NaCl) or the antagonist alone given 60 minutes prior to the activity test. Hatched bars represent activity measured 20 minutes following the injection of 5.0 mg/kg TFMPP. (*) indicates that treatment with TFMPP reduced activity significantly compared with saline, according to Student's t-test, $p < 0.05$. Pretreatment with the nonselective 5-HT antagonist metergoline (0.3 mg/kg) or the 5-HT1C/2 antagonist mianserin (5.0 mg/kg) prevented TFMPP from producing significant reductions of locomotor activity. In contrast, pretreatment with the 5-HT1A/1B antagonist pindolol (10 mg/kg) or the 5-HT2 antagonist ketanserin (10 mg/kg) failed to prevent the effect of TFMPP on locomotor activity. These results indicate that TFMPP's ability to suppress locomotor activity may be associated with stimulation of the 5-HT1C receptor.

were unable to block TFMPP's effects on behavior (Fig. 5.4) even though they prevented 8-OH-DPAT's ability to cause the 5-HT syndrome (cf. Fig. 5.2).

In contrast, increases in locomotor activity of rats or mice caused by the piperidinyl indole agonist RU 24969 have been proposed as a behavioral model for the activation of 5-HT$_{1B}$ receptors (Green, Guy, & Gardner, 1984) because this agonist has slight selectivity for 5-HT$_{1B}$ receptors (Lucki et al., 1987a; Sills et al., 1984). However, the hyperactivity caused by RU 24969 may also be mediated by catecholamine systems because this effect is blocked by pretreatment with catecholamine antagonists such as prazosin or pimozide (Lucki et al., 1987a; Tricklebank, Middlemiss, & Neill, 1986).

Head Shaking Behavior

Most mammalian species exhibit spontaneous head shaking behavior. This behavior appears as a rapid rhythmic shaking of the head in a radial motion (for review, see Handley & Singh, 1986a), and resembles in form a reflex elicited by stimulating the external auditory meatus. The response is also known as "wet-dog shakes" or called a head twitch in mice. Administration to rodents of a variety of drugs that stimulate 5-HT receptors increase spontaneous head and body shaking behavior (Bedard & Pycock, 1977; Corne, Pickering, & Warner, 1963). In rats prominent head shaking behavior accompanied by body shakes is produced by 5-HTP in combination with carbidopa pretreatment (Bedard & Pycock, 1977; Lucki et al., 1984), or by 5-HT precursors when combined with a 5-HT uptake inhibitor (Arnt, Hyttel, & Larsen, 1984). 5-HT agonists, such as quipazine, and more selective 5-HT$_2$ agonists, such as mescaline, DOB or DOI, also produce head shaking behavior in rats (Lucki et al., 1984; Niemegeers et al., 1983; Vetulani, Bednarczyk, Reichenberg, & Rokosz, 1980; Wieland & Lucki, unpublished data). However, 5-HT agonists that are selective for other receptor subtypes, such as 5-MeODMT, 8-OH-DPAT, TFMPP, or m-CPP, do not produce reliable head shaking behavior in rats (Lucki, unpublished data).

The head shaking response caused by 5-HT agonists is associated with the activation of 5-HT$_2$ receptors. Head shaking behavior caused by 5-HTP in mice or rats is blocked by a variety of nonselective 5-HT antagonists, such as metergoline, methysergide, and mianserin, as well as by 5-HT$_2$-selective antagonists such as ketanserin, pipamperone, or pirenperone. The potency of the antagonists to block 5-HT-mediated shaking behavior correlates with their affinity for the 5-HT$_2$ receptor (Colpaert & Janssen, 1983; Lucki et al., 1984; Niemegeers et al., 1983; Ogren et al., 1979; Peroutka, Lebovitz, & Snyder, 1981). The potent ability of the 5-HT$_2$ antagonist ketanserin to block the head shake response (ED50 = 0.1 mg/kg; Lucki et al., 1984; Lucki, Eberle, & Minugh-Purvis, 1987a) taken together with the inability of ketanserin to block the 5-HT syndrome up to doses of 20 mg/kg (Lucki et al., 1984; present study) represents an impressive demonstration of the selective behavioral effects of this compound. 5-HT antagonists block 5-HT-stimulated head shaking behavior without altering reflex activity elicited by mechanical stimulation of the aural pinnae (Corne et al., 1963; Lucki, Eberle, & Minugh-Purvis, 1987a). Although other drugs such as opiates, thyrotropin releasing hormone, and carbachol also cause head shaking in rodents (see Handley & Singh, 1986a), they do not appear to cause their effects at 5-HT receptors (Bedard & Pycock, 1977; Drust & Conner, 1983). In addition to 5-HT antagonists, however, alterations of other neurotransmitter systems may affect 5-HT-mediated shaking behavior. For example, the alpha$_2$ adrenergic agonists clonidine and guanabenz inhibit 5-HT-mediated shaking (Handley & Brown, 1982; Matthews & Smith, 1980) perhaps because these drugs inhibit the pinnae reflex (Brown & Handley, 1980). There are conflicting reports that lesions of noradrenergic neurons result in increases (Heal, Philpot, O'Shaughnessy, & Davis, 1986), decreases (Handley & Singh, 1986b), or no change (Bednarczyk & Vetulani, 1978) in 5-HT-mediated shaking behavior.

The ability of acute administration of antidepressant drugs to alter 5-HT-mediated head shaking behavior has consistently implicated 5-HT among their possible mechanisms of action. For example, the ability of MAOIs and 5-HT uptake inhibitors, such as fluoxetine, to potentiate head shaking behavior caused by 5-HT precursors agrees with the ability of these drugs to enhance 5-HT neurotransmission in *vivo* (Arnt et al., 1984; Matthews & Smith, 1980). However, a number of antidepressants, such as amitriptyline, nortriptyline, mianserin and trazadone, were first suggested to be 5-HT antagonists because they inhibited 5-HT-related shaking behavior (Fuxe, Ogren, Agnati, Gustafson, & Jonsson, 1977; Maj, Palider, & Rawlow, 1979; Ogren et al., 1979). Subsequently, these drugs were shown to be potent direct antagonists of 5-HT_2 receptors (Peroutka et al., 1981).

REGULATION OF BEHAVIORAL RESPONSES ELICITED BY 5-HT AGONISTS

The previous section described behavioral responses elicited by stimulating different types of 5-HT receptors. These responses can serve as indices to measure functional changes associated with specific 5-HT receptor subtypes that are produced by different treatments that change the availability of 5-HT content and the role of 5-HT receptors in mediating such effects. Although some of these treatments have been examined previously using nonselective agonists, this section reviews our more recent studies that have used selective 5-HT agonists to elicit the behavioral responses.

Destruction of 5-HT Neurons

A large body of data indicates that behavioral supersensitivity to 5-HT agonists develops after lesions to central serotonergic pathways (for review, see Frazer, Offord, & Lucki, 1988). The different unconditioned behaviors elicited by selective 5-HT agonists have been examined following the destruction of 5-HT neurons by the intraventricular administration of the neurotoxin 5,7-dihydroxytryptamine (5,7-DHT) in rats pretreated with desipramine to prevent the destruction of noradrenergic neurons. This treatment caused 84% depletion of forebrain 5-HT content without significant alteration of the content of norepinephrine and dopamine.

Behavioral activity associated with each of the different 5-HT receptor subtypes was determined by measuring the ability of different agonists to produce their characteristic behavioral effects. The behaviors examined were: (1) the 5-HT behavioral syndrome produced by the 5-HT$_{1A}$ agonist 8-OH-DPAT; (2) reduction of locomotor activity produced by the 5-HT$_{1B/1C}$ agonist m-CPP; and (3) head shaking behavior produced by the 5-HT$_2$ agonist DOB. The results are presented in Table 5.2 as the dose required to produce a half-maximal behavioral effect (ED50) in rats treated with either 5,7-DHT or vehicle. 5,7-DHT treatment increased the potency of each of the selective 5-HT agonists, as revealed by a 2–4 fold parallel shift to the left for causing each of the behavioral responses. That 5-HT neuronal destruction potentiated the behavioral response to each agonist indicates that these agonists cause their behavioral effects by actions at 5-HT receptors located postsynaptically. Furthermore, the relatively similar magnitude of change in potency of the agonists may indicate a relatively similar degree of supersensitivity to direct activation of each of these receptor subtypes following the destruction of 5-HT neurons.

Relatively few studies have examined whether 5-HT neuronal destruction produces changes in 5-HT receptors using selective radioligands. However, thus far, little support exists that increases in 5-HT receptor density are produced following 5-HT neuronal destruction (see Frazer et al., 1988). Therefore, other mechanisms must be studied in order to account for the common finding of enhanced behavioral responses to 5-HT agonists following denervation of 5-HT neurons.

Chronic Administration of 5-HT Agonists

It is generally known that the repeated administration of agonists produces a gradual reduction in their effects, which is called tolerance. Tolerance develops to a number of the behavioral effects of 5-HT agonists following their repeated administration (see Frazer et al., 1988). However, few studies have examined

TABLE 5.2
Increased Sensitivity to Behavioral Responses Elicited
by Selective Serotonin Agonists Following Treatment
with 5,7-dihydroxytryptamine

	ED50 for Eliciting Response (mg/kg)		
Behavior (Agonist)	Control	5,7-DHT	Increase in Sensitivity
5-HT Syndrome (8-OH-DPAT)	1.9	1.0	1.9
Reduction of activity (m-CPP)	1.4	0.35	4.0
Head Shaking Behavior (± DOB)	0.52	0.28	1.9

whether the development of tolerance to a behavioral response mediated by one 5-HT receptor is accompanied by tolerance to behaviors mediated by other 5-HT receptors. In one such study, the ability of chronic administration of two 5-HT agonists that cause different behavioral responses to produce tolerance to their own behavioral effects and cross-tolerance to the behavioral response of the other agonist was examined (Sills, Lucki, & Frazer, 1985). Chronic administration of m-CPP for 14 days produced tolerance to its activity-reducing effects but failed to alter the ability of 5-MeODMT to produce the 5-HT syndrome. Conversely, tolerance to the behavioral effect caused by 5-MeODMT was produced by its repeated administration for 14 days without causing cross-tolerance to m-CPP's activity-suppressant effects.

This study was recently extended by us to examine whether chronic administration of selective 5-HT agonists would produce cross-tolerance to the same behavioral response caused by a different agonist. These results are shown in Fig. 5.5. Chronic administration of 8-OH-DPAT (2 mg/kg tid for 14 days) produced a 3-fold shift to the right of the dose-effect curve for 5-MeODMT to produce the 5-HT behavioral syndrome. However, these rats demonstrated no change in the ability of m-CPP to reduce locomotor activity. Conversely, chronic administration of TFMPP (5 mg/kg tid for 17 days) reduced the sensitivity to m-CPP-induced reductions of locomotor activity by 2-fold but did not alter the ability of 8-OH-DPAT to produce the 5-HT behavioral syndrome. These data are consistent with mediation and regulation of these behavioral effects by different 5-HT receptor subtypes.

Chronic Administration of Antidepressant Drugs

Particular interest has focused on the effects of chronic antidepressant treatments on 5-HT-mediated behavioral responses (see Frazer et al., 1988) because they have prominent effects on 5-HT neurons when administered acutely, either by inhibiting the uptake of 5-HT, inhibiting the metabolism of 5-HT by MAO, or by being antagonists at 5-HT_2 receptors (see Frazer & Conway, 1984). Patients usually must take antidepressant medications for several weeks before reporting therapeutic effects.

The 5-HT behavioral syndrome caused by the agonists 5-MeODMT or LSD was prevented following the repeated administration of monoamine oxidase inhibitors (MAOIs) such as nialamide, phenelzine, or pargyline to rats for 7 days (Lucki & Frazer, 1982a). Acute administration of the MAOIs failed to change the ability of the agonists to elicit the syndrome. In contrast, chronic treatment with the tricyclic antidepressants desipramine, amitriptyline, chlorimipramine, or the atypical antidepresant iprindole failed to alter the ability of 5-MeODMT to cause the syndrome. The ability of chronic MAOI treatment to block the appearance of the 5-HT syndrome is probably caused by a persistent overexposure of postsynatpic 5-HT_{1A} receptors to endogenous 5-HT. Prior depletion of 5-HT

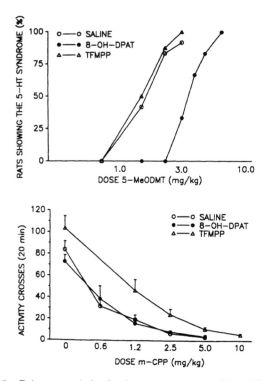

FIG. 5.5. Tolerance to behavioral responses produced by 5-HT receptor stimulation following the chronic administration of agonists selective for 5-HT receptor subtypes. Separate groups of rats were given the following treatments: Saline (N = 60); the 5-HT$_{1A}$ agonist 8-OH-DPAT (2.0 mg/kg tid; N = 30); or the 5-HT$_{1B/1C}$ agonist TFMPP (5.0 mg/kg tid; N = 40). *Upper panel:* The ability of 5-MeODMT to produce the 5-HT syndrome in rats treated chronically with the 5-HT agonists for 14 days. The 5-HT syndrome was rated as described previously (see Fig. 5.1). Each point represents values from separate groups of rats: Saline, N = 12; 8-OH-DPAT, N = 6; and TFMPP, N = 8. Tolerance was produced to the effects of 5-MeODMT only in the group treated chronically with 8-OH-DPAT. *Lower panel:* The ability of m-CPP to reduce the locomotor activity of rats treated chronically with 5-HT agonists for 17 days. Activity was measured as described previously in Figure 4. Each point represents mean activity values from separate groups of rats: Saline, N = 12; 8-OH-DPAT, N = 6; TFMPP, N = 8. Tolerance was produced only in the group treated chronically with TFMPP.

content using PCPA or the destruction of 5-HT neurons using 5,7-DHT prevents chronic MAOI administration from blocking the 5-HT syndrome (Lucki & Frazer, 1982a; Lucki & Press, unpublished).

Similar to the 5-HT syndrome, the suppression of locomotor activity produced by the $5\text{-HT}_{1B/1C}$ agonist m-CPP is attenuated following repeated, but not by acute, administration of the MAOIs phenelzine or nialamide (Lucki & Frazer, 1985). In contrast, chronic treatment with other antidepressants such as amitriptyline, desipramine or iprindole did not alter this behavioral effect of m-CPP.

In contrast to the 5-HT behavioral syndrome and locomotor activity, hypothermia produced in mice by the 5-HT_{1A} agonist 8-OH-DPAT is reduced following the chronic administration of the tricyclic antidepressants amitriptyline or desipramine, the atypical antidepressants zimelidine or mianserin, and by the MAOI tranylcypromine (Goodwin, De Souza, & Green, 1985b, 1987b). Repeated application of electroconvulsive shock to mice or rats also diminished DPAT-induced hypothermia (Goodwin et al., 1985b; 1987b). As the hypothermic effect of 8-OH-DPAT may be mediated by presynatpic 5-HT_{1A} receptors, antidepressant drug treatments could produce different effects at 5-HT_{1A} receptors located either presynaptically or postsynaptically.

Studies examining head shaking behavior produced by 5-HT precursors or by 5-HT agonists have reported both increases and decreases in the magnitude of this response following chronic antidepressant drug treatments. In general, however, studies that measured head shaking behavior 24 hours or less following the last treatment dose reported a reduction of this behavioral response following chronic treatment with either tricyclics, atypicals, or MAOI antidepressants (see Frazer et al., 1988). Since chronic administration of antidepressant drugs reduces the density of 5-HT_2 receptors measured in rat frontal cortex (Lucki & Frazer, 1985; Peroutka & Snyder, 1980), the diminished head shaking response to 5-HT agonists is generally consistent with this effect. In contrast, repeated electoconvulsive shock treatment to rats increases head shaking caused by 5-HT agonists and also increases the density of 5-HT_2 receptors (Lebrecht & Nowak, 1980; Vetulani, Lebrecht, & Pilc, 1981). However, most studies have measured the changes in 5-HT_2 receptors caused by antidepressant drugs only in rat frontal cortex, the site of their greatest density. Because the 5-HT-mediated head shaking response is probably not mediated by receptors located in the frontal cortex (Bedard & Pycock, 1977; Lucki & Minugh-Purvis, 1987), it will be important to measure receptor changes in the brain area responsible for this behavior (or any behavior) when studying receptor correlates of behavior changes caused by antidepressant drugs.

The ability of chronic administration of a variety of antidepressant drugs to alter 5-HT-mediated responses in rats was reexamined using selective 5-HT agonists (see Table 5.3). Chronic administration of either phenelzine (10 mg/kg once daily for 7 days), desipramine, or imipramine (10 mg/kg bid for 14 days) to rats diminished the hypothermic effect of 8-OH-DPAT. In contrast, only chronic

TABLE 5.3
Altered Behavioral Responses to 5-HT Agonists Following Chronic Treatment
with Antidepressant Drugs

Antidepressant Drug (Treatment)	5-HT-Mediated Response/Agonist		
	5-HT Syndrome[c] 8-OH-DPAT	Hypothermia[d] 8-OH-DPAT	Head Shakes[e] DOB
Saline	94% (16/17)	−2.24 ± .21	23.3 ± 2.0
Phenelzine (10 mg/kg once daily for 7 days)	11% (1/9)[b]	−0.55 ± .33[a]	5.7 ± 2.0[a]
Desipramine (10 mg/kg bid for 14 days)	75% (6/8)	−0.53 ± .32[a]	16.9 ± 2.8[a]
Imipramine (10 mg/kg bid for 14 days)	71% (5/7)	−1.28 ± .34[a]	14.8 ± 3.3[a]

[a]Value differs significantly from corresponding value in saline-treated rats, $p <$ 0.05.

[b]Value differs significantly from corresponding value in saline-treated rats, according to chi-square test, $p < 0.05$.

[c]The 5-HT syndrome was assessed in rats after administration of 4.0 mg/kg 8-OH-DPAT. Values are expressed as the % of animals showing the 5-HT syndrome as determined by the presence of 4 out of 6 critical symptoms (Lucki et al., 1984), and the values in parentheses indicate the number of rats showing the syndrome/the number of rats tested.

[d]Hypothermia was determined as the change in rectal temperature measured 30 minutes after administration of 4.0 mg/kg 8-OH-DPAT to rats. Values are expressed as the mean change in degrees C from baseline ± 1 SEM.

[e]Head shaking behavior was determined as the number of head shakes measured for 30 min after administration of 1.0 mg/kg DOB. Values are expressed as the mean total shakes ± 1 SEM.

administration of phenelzine blocked the 5-HT behavioral syndrome (Table 5.3), in agreement with our previous study using other agonists to produce this behavioral response (Lucki & Frazer, 1982a). Thus, the hypothermic effect of 8-OH-DPAT, which may be mediated by presynaptic 5-HT$_{1A}$ receptors, may be commonly inhibited by a number of antidepressant treatments whereas the 5-HT behavioral syndrome, mediated by postsynaptic 5-HT$_{1A}$ receptors, was blocked only by chronic MAOI administration. In addition, chronic administration of the tricyclic and MAOI antidepressant drugs commonly reduced the ability of the maximally effective dose of the selective 5-HT$_2$ agonist DOB (1.0 mg/kg) to produce head shaking behavior when this effect was measured 24 hours following the last drug treatment (Table 5.3). These observations that 5-HT-mediated behavioral responses are altered following chronic antidepressant drug treatments support the idea that changes in serotonergic systems, particularly presynaptic 5-HT$_{1A}$ and 5-HT$_2$ receptors, may be important to the therapeutic effects of antidepressant drugs.

DRUG DISCRIMINATION STUDIES

Recently drug discrimination procedures have been used as a functional assay for selective 5-HT agonists. Drug discrimination procedures require animals to emit one response when administered a drug and a different response when no drug or other drugs are administered (for description, see Overton, 1987). Following extensive training to discriminate the presence versus the absence of drug, a number of different types of studies can be conducted. For example, in drug substitution tests, different doses of drugs other than the training drug are administered to determine if rats will make the response reinforced under the training drug. Drugs that produce responding resembling the training drug are said to generalize to the training stimulus. The potency relationship among a number of agonists with varying affinity for 5-HT receptor subtypes can be studied. Animals may also be pretreated with selective 5-HT receptor antagonists in order to determine if they block the stimulus effects of the training drug. This type of drug discrimination experiment in animals may be analogous to studies of the subjective effects of drugs produced in human subjects (Schuster, Fischman, & Johanson, 1981).

A large number of studies have employed 5-HT agonists as training drugs in drug discrimination studies (for review, see Glennon & Lucki, 1988). More recent studies have used agonists that binding studies identified to be selective for 5-HT receptor subtypes. In general, such studies indicate that the stimulus properties of 5-HT agonists may form distinct groupings based upon the training drug's affinity for subtypes of 5-HT receptors.

The demonstration that 8-hydroxy-2(di-n-propylamino)tetralin (8-OH-DPAT) binds selectively to central $5-HT_{1A}$ sites (Middlemiss & Fozard, 1983) provided an important tool for examining behavioral effects that were caused by stimulation of $5-HT_{1A}$ receptor. Several groups have now shown that 8-OH-DPAT serves as an effective training compound in drug discrimination studies (Cunningham, Callahan, & Appel, 1987; Glennon, 1986a; Lucki, 1988; Tricklebank, Neill, Kidd, & Fozard, 1987). Agonists that are selective for other 5-HT receptor subtypes, such as TFMPP and m-CPP ($5-HT_{1B}$ and $5-HT_{1C}$) or DOM and DOI ($5-HT_2$), do not substitute for the 8-OH-DPAT stimulus cue. Pretreatment with a variety of antagonists including $5-HT_2$ antagonists ketanserin and pirenperone and the $5-HT_3$ antagonist MDL 72222 failed to block the 8-OH-DPAT stimulus up to doses that caused a general disruption of responding. However, pretreatment with $(-)$pindolol or $(-)$alprenolol, antagonists with high affinity for $5-HT_{1A}$ receptors in addition to their beta-adrenergic antagonist effects, blocked the stimulus effects of 8-OH-DPAT (Tricklebank et al., 1987). Recently, potent and selective affinity for the $5-HT_{1A}$ receptor has been identified for drugs such as busipirone, gepirone and ipsapirone. These drugs are used to treat anxiety disorders in humans (Goldberg & Finnerty, 1979). They also cause behavioral effects in animals typical of antianxiety agents but not by the activation of benzodiazepine receptors (Eison, Eison, Stanley, & Riblet, 1986). Rats trained to discriminate the stimulus properties of 8-OH-DPAT demonstrate generaliza-tion to these nonbenzodiazepine anxiolytic agents that are selective for the 5-HT_{1A} receptor subtype (Cunningham et al., 1987; Glennon, 1986a; Tricklebank et al., 1987). When buspirone or ipsapirone is used as the training drug, their stimulus effects generalize to 8-OH-DPAT but not to benzodiazepine anxiolytics (Mansbach & Barrett, 1987; Spencer & Traber, 1987). These studies support the idea that the stimulus effects of these anxiolytic drugs involve a 5-HT_{1A} mecha-nism that may be involved in producing their therapeutic effects.

The stimulus effects of TFMPP generalize to other compounds that display modest selectivity for the 5-HT_{1B} receptor, such as m-CPP and RU 24969 (Cunningham & Appel, 1986; Lucki, 1988; McKenney & Glennon, 1986). The stimulus effects of TFMPP do not generalize to 5-HT_{1A} selective agonists such as 8-OH-DPAT, buspirone, ipsapirone, or gepirone nor to 5-HT_2-selective ago-nists such as DOM, DOB, or DOI. Presently, no antagonists have been identified that completely block the TFMPP stimulus, although pindolol, propranolol and mesulergine have been reported to substitute for TFMPP (Glennon, Pierson, & McKenney, 1988).

The stimulus effects of drugs that are hallucinogenic in humans, including indolealkylamines such as LSD and phenylalkylamines such as DOM, DOB and DOI, appear to involve stimulation of the 5-HT_2 receptor. Rats trained to dis-criminate the stimulus effects of hallucinogens, such as DOM or LSD, respond to a variety of other hallucinogenic drugs as if the training drug were adminis-tered (Colpaert, Meert, Niemegeers, & Janssen, 1985; Glennon, Young, & Rosecrans, 1983). The derived ED50 values of drugs that generalize to the DOM stimulus is correlated with their hallucinogenic potency in man (Glennon et al., 1984). However, the stimulus effects of 5-HT_2-selective agonists, such as DOM or DOI, do not generalize to agonists that are selective for other 5-HT receptor subtypes such as 8-OH-DPAT, TFMPP, or RU 24969 (Glennon, 1986b; Glen-non & Hauck, 1985). Furthermore, studies using DOM as a discriminative stimulus have shown that its effects are blocked by a variety of agonists that commonly block the 5-HT_2 receptor, including ketanserin, ritanserin, and LY 53857 (Glennon et al., 1983; Glennon & Hauck, 1985). The stimulus effects of LSD are also blocked by selective 5-HT_2 antagonists (Colpaert et al., 1985; Cunningham & Appel, 1987).

5-HT RECEPTOR SUBTYPES AND BEHAVIOR

Studies of unconditioned behaviors elicited by 5-HT agonists and the stimulus properties of 5-HT agonists using drug discrimination have provided good evi-dence that the functional effects of 5-HT agonists depend on their affinity for distinct 5-HT receptor subtypes. A further goal of behavioral research is to identify the involvement of 5-HT receptors in natural behavioral functions.

Using behavioral models of 5-HT receptor activation as a guide, a number of studies have begun to assess the role of 5-HT in such behaviors, such as arousal, feeding behavior, sexual behavior, and aggression (see Glennon & Lucki, 1988). Some of these effects are summarized in Table 5.4.

The startle reflex has been used as a method for examining the effects of 5-HT-related drugs on modulating the behavioral response to external stimuli. The administration of 5-HT agonists that differ in their selectivity for 5-HT receptors affect the startle response in different ways. For example, systemic administra-

TABLE 5.4
Proposed Behavioral Functions Associated with
Different 5-HT Receptor Subtypes

I. 5-HT$_{1A}$ Receptor
A. Presynaptic:
Antipunishment effect
Hypothermia
Increased feeding behavior
Facilitation of ejaculation

B. Postsynaptic:
5-HT behavioral syndrome

C. Localization not yet established:
Stimulus effects of 8-OH-DPAT and atypical anxiolytic drugs
Facilitation of startle reflex
Inhibition of female sexual receptivity
Behavioral response to stressors

II. 5-HT$_{1B}$ Receptor
Increased locomotor activity by RU 24969
Decreased feeding behavior by RU 24969
Stimulus effects of TFMPP (?)

III. 5-HT$_{1C}$ Receptor
Decreased locomotor activity by TFMPP and m-CPP
Decreased feeding behavior by TFMPP and m-CPP
Stimulus effects of TFMPP (?)

IV. 5-HT$_2$ Receptor
Stimulus effects of hallucinogenic drugs
Hyperthermia by MK 212
Head shaking behavior or head twitches
Tryptamine-induced convulsions

V. 5-HT$_3$ Receptor
Anti-emesis (peripheral effect)
Anxiety (speculated central effect)
Psychosis (speculated central effect)

---

tion of the 5-HT_{1A} agonist 8-OH-DPAT enhances the acoustic startle reflex (Davis, Cassella, Wren, & Kehne, 1986; Svensson & Ahlenius, 1983), the $5\text{-HT}_{1B/1C}$ agonist m-CPP suppresses the startle response (Davis et al., 1986), and mescaline enhances acoustic startle by stimulating the 5-HT_2 receptor (Davis, 1987). Further studies suggest that different sites in the CNS may be involved in these effects. For example, 8-OH-DPAT elevated startle when administered onto the spinal cord but not intraventricularly, whereas m-CPP depressed startle when given intraventricularly but not intrathecally (Davis et al., 1986). Future work is well-positioned to examine precisely how 5-HT agonists modulate the primary startle circuit (Davis, Gendelman, Tischler, & Gendelman, 1982).

Studies of deprivation-induced feeding behavior have shown that agonists that are selective for the 5-HT_{1A} receptor (8-OH-DPAT; Bendotti & Samanin, 1987); 5-HT_{1B} receptor (RU 24969; Bendotti & Samanin, 1987), the $5\text{-HT}_{1B/1C}$ receptor (m-CPP and TFMPP; Fuller et al., 1981; Samanin et al., 1979), and 5-HT_2 receptor (DOI; Schechter & Simansky, 1988) can inhibit deprivation-induced food consumption. More detailed behavioral analyses may reveal how the anorexic effects of these drugs differ. It is also not known whether activation of these 5-HT receptors are involved in controlling natural feeding behavior or the regulation of body weight.

The 5-HT_{1A}-selective agonist 8-OH-DPAT produces different effects on sexual behavior in male and female rats. Male sexual behaviors, such as mounting and ejaculation frequency, are increased by 8-OH-DPAT (Ahlenius et al., 1981; Mendelson & Gorzalka, 1986), whereas the lordosis response in female rats is inhibited by 8-OH-DPAT (Ahlenius, Fernandez-Guasti, Hjorth, & Larsson, 1986; Mendelson & Gorzalka, 1986). Different roles for activation of other 5-HT receptors in sexual behavior have also been suggested (see Mendelson & Gorzalka, 1989).

The clinical use of buspirone for generalized anxiety disorder and the development of its congeners gepirone and ipsapirone for anxiety and depression has created interest in the role of 5-HT systems in the pharmacology of these atypical psychotherapeutic drugs. These drugs, along with 8-OH-DPAT are active in preclinical behavioral screening tests for both anxiety (Eison et al., 1986; Engel et al., 1984) and for depression (Cervo & Samanin, 1987; Kennett, Dourish, & Curzon, 1987). These behavioral effects may provide functional models for determining how buspirone and its analogs produce their therapeutic effects in affective disorders.

SUMMARY

The consistent demonstration that 5-HT agonists and antagonists produce specific effects according to their affinity for 5-HT receptor subtypes provides evidence that the different types of 5-HT receptors must be considered a mechanism controlling the behavioral functions served by 5-HT. Dually, these studies show that the different populations of receptors defined using radioligand binding techniques are relevant for understanding 5-HT's physiological roles in the CNS. Concerning present clinical applications, the affinity of buspirone and associated compounds for the 5-HT$_{1A}$ receptor has created a new class of drugs that are being evaluated for therapeutic efficacy for anxiety and depression. The hallucinogenic effects of DOM, LSD, mescaline and related drugs appear to involve the selective activation of 5-HT$_2$ receptors. The ability of a variety of antidepressant drugs to reduce the density of 5-HT$_2$ receptors may be important to their therapeutic effects. The role of selective 5-HT agonists and antagonists is now being reconsidered for behavioral functions and in clinical applications that were formerly associated loosely with 5-HT in a nonselective manner.

There are serious limitations in specificity to most of the 5-HT agonists and antagonists presently available and rapid advances in 5-HT pharmacology often complicate the interpretation of studies (see Fozard, 1987). However, careful pharmacological procedures, such as the use of potency relationships among agonists or antagonists, the comparison between active and inactive stereoisomers, and studying the effects of families of compounds instead of just a single prototypic drug, help to ensure that behavioral investigations of 5-HT-related compounds provide important information regardless of changes required in 5-HT receptor terminology. There is no question that the development of more selective and specific agonists and antagonists for established 5-HT receptors than those presently available is required for further progress in this area. Some investigators have used radioligand binding techniques to propose additional classes of 5-HT receptors from identified binding sites. These developments in 5-HT pharmacology are exciting but need not deter behavioral research since the significance of these binding sites will remain questionable until selective agonists and antagonists are identified to determine the site's functional importance. Once these compounds become available, however, behavioral research will necessarily guide the physiological analysis of how these compounds exert their functional effects in the CNS and in the assessment of their potential usefulness in medicine.

ACKNOWLEDGMENTS

The author's research presented in this chapter was supported by USPHS grants MH 36262 and GM 34781.

REFERENCES

Ahlenius, S., Fernandez-Guasti, A., Hjorth, S., & Larsson, K. (1986). Suppression of lordosis behavior by the putative 5-HT receptor agonist 8-OH-DPAT in the rat. *European Journal of Pharmacology, 124,* 361–363.

Ahlenius, S., Larsson, K., Svensson, L., Hjorth, S., Carlsson, A., Lindberg, P., Wilstrom, H., Sanchez, D., Arvidsson, L.-E., Hacksell, U., & Nilsson, J. L. G. (1981). Effects of a new type of 5-HT receptor agonist on male rat sexual behavior. *Pharmacology, Biochemistry, and Behavior, 15*, 785–792.

Arnt, J., Hyttel, J., & Larsen, J. J. (1984). The citalopram/5-HTP-induced head shake syndrome is correlated to 5-HT$_2$ receptor affinity and also influenced by other transmitters. *Acta Pharmacologica et Toxicology, 55*, 363–372.

Asarch, K. B., Ransom, R. W., & Shih, J. C. (1985). 5-HT-1a and 5-HT-1b selectivity of two phenylpiperazine derivatives: Evidence for 5-HT1b heterogeneity. *Life Sciences, 36*, 1265–1273.

Azmitia, E. C. (1987). The CNS serotonergic system: Progression toward a collaborative organization. In H. Y. Meltzer (Ed.), *Psychopharmacology: The third generation of progress* (pp. 61–73). New York: Raven Press.

Bedard, P., & Pycock, C. J. (1977). "Wet-dog" shake behaviour in the rat: A possible quantitative model of central 5-hydroxytryptamine activity. *Neuropharmacology, 16*, 663–670.

Bednarczyk, B., & Vetulani, J. (1978). Antagonism of clonidine to shaking behaviour in morphine abstinence syndrome and to head-twitches produced by serotonergic agents in the rat. *Polish Journal of Pharmacology and Pharmacy, 30*, 307–322.

Bendotti, C., & Samanin, R. (1987). The role of putative 5-HT$_{1A}$ and 5-HT$_{1B}$ receptors in the control of feeding in rats. *Life Sciences, 41*, 635–642.

Bradley, P. B., Engel, G., Feniuk, W., Fozard, J. R., Humphrey, P. P. A., Middlemiss, D. N., Mylecharane, E. J., Richardson, B. P., & Saxena, P. R. (1986). Proposals for the classification and nomenclature of functional receptors for 5-hydroxytryptamine. *Neuropharmacology, 25*, 563–576.

Brown, J., & Handley, S. L. (1980). Effects on the pinna reflex of drugs acting at alpha-adrenoceptors. *Journal of Pharmacy and Pharmacology, 32*, 436–437.

Cervo, L., & Samanin, R. (1987). Potential antidepressant properties of 8-hydroxy-2-(di-n-propylamino)tetralin, a selective serotonin$_{1A}$ receptor agonist. *European Journal of Pharmacology, 144*, 223–229.

Colpaert, F. C., & Janssen, P. A. J. (1983). The head-twitch response to intraperitoneal injection of 5-hydroxytryptophan in the rat: Antagonist effects of purported 5-hydroxytryptamine antagonists and of pirenperone, an LSD antagonist. *Neuropharmacology, 22*, 993–1000.

Colpaert, F. C., Meert, T. F., Niemegeers, C. J. E., & Janssen, P. A. J. (1985). Behavioral and 5-HT antagonist effects of ritanserin: A pure and selective antagonist of LSD discrimination in rat. *Psychopharmacology, 86*, 45–54.

Conn, P. J., & Sanders-Bush, E. (1987). Relative efficacies of piperazines at the phosphoinositide hydrolysis-linked serotonergic (5-HT-2 and 5-HT1c) receptors. *Journal of Pharmacology and Experimental Therapeutics, 242*, 552–557.

Corne, S. J., Pickering, R. W., & Warner, B. T. (1963). A method for assessing the effect of drugs on the central actions of 5-hydroxytryptamine. *British Journal of Pharmacology, 20*, 106–120.

Cunningham, K. A., & Appel, J. B. (1986). Possible 5-hydroxytryptamine$_1$ (5-HT$_1$) receptor involvement in the stimulus properties of 1-(m-trifluoromethylphenyl)piperazine (TFMPP). *Journal of Pharmacology and Experimental Therapeutics, 237*, 369–377.

Cunningham, K. A., & Appel, J. B. (1987). Neuropharmacological reassessment of the discriminative stimulus properties of d-lysergic acid diethylamide (LSD). *Psychopharmacology, 91*, 67–73.

Cunningham, K. A., Callahan, P. M., & Appel, J. B. (1987). Discriminative stimulus properties of 8-hydroxy-2-(di-n-propylamino)tetralin (8-OHDPAT): Implications for understanding the actions of novel anxiolytics. *European Journal of Pharmacology, 138*, 29–36.

Davis, M. (1987). Mescaline: Excitatory effects on acoustic startle are blocked by serotonin$_2$ antagonists. *Psychopharmacology, 93*, 286–291.

Davis, M., Astrachan, D. I., & Kass, E. (1980). Excitatory and inhibitory effects of serotonin on sensorimotor reactivity measured with acoustic startle. *Science, 209*, 521–523.

Davis, M., Cassella, J. V., Wren, W. H., & Kehne, J. H. (1986). Serotonin receptor subtype agonists: Differential effects on sensorimotor reactivity measured with acoustic startle. *Psychopharmacology Bulletin, 22,* 837–843.

Davis, M., Gendelman, D. S., Tischler, M. D., & Gendelman, P. M. (1982). A primary acoustic startle circuit: Lesion and stimulation studies. *Journal of Neuroscience, 2,* 791–805.

Deakin, J. F. W., & Dashwood, M. R. (1981). The differential neurochemical bases of the behaviours elicited by serotonergic agents and by the combination of a monoamine oxidase inhibitor and L-DOPA. *Neuropharmacology, 20,* 123–130.

Deakin, J. F. W., & Green, A. R. (1978). The effect of putative 5-hydroxytryptamine antagonists on the behaviour produced by the administration of tranylcypromine and L-tryptophan or tranylcypromine and L-dopa to rats. *British Journal of Pharmacology, 64,* 201–209.

Dickinson, S. L., Jackson, A., & Curzon, G. (1983). Effect of apomorphine on behavior induced by 5-methoxy-N,N-dimethyltryptamine: Three different scoring methods give three different conclusions. *Psychopharmacology, 80,* 196–197.

Drust, E. G., & Connor, J. E. (1983). Pharmacological analysis of shaking behavior induced by enkephalins, thyrotropin-releasing hormone or serotonin in rats: Evidence for different mechanisms. *Journal of Pharmacology and Experimental Therapeutics, 224,* 148–154.

Eison, A. S., Eison, M. S., Stanley, M., & Riblet, L. A. (1986). Serotonergic mechanisms in the behavioral effects of buspirone and gepirone. *Pharmacology, Biochemistry and Behavior, 24,* 701–707.

Engel, G., Gothert, M., Hoyer, D., Schlicker, E., & Hillenbrand, K. (1986). Identity of inhibitory presynaptic 5-hydroxytryptamine (5-HT) autoreceptors in the rat brain cortex with 5-HT-1B binding sites. *Naunyn-Schmiedeberg's Archives of Pharmacology, 332,* 1–7.

Engel, J. A., Hjorth, S., Svenson, K., Carlsson, A., & Liljequist, S. (1984). Anticonflict effect of the putative serotonin receptor agonist 8-hydroxy-2-(di-n-propylamino)tetralin (8-OH-DPAT). *European Journal of Pharmacology, 105,* 365–368.

Fozard, J. R. (1987). 5-HT: The enigma variations. *Trends in Pharmacological Sciences, 8,* 501–506.

Frazer, A., & Conway, P. (1984). Pharmacologic mechanisms of action of antidepressant. *Psychiatric Clinics of North America, 7,* 575–586.

Frazer, A., Offord, S. J., & Lucki, I. (1988). Regulation of serotonin receptor and responsiveness in the brain. In E. Sanders-Bush (Ed.), *The serotonin receptors* (pp. 319–362). Clifton, NJ: Humana.

Fuller, R. W., Snoddy, H. D., Mason, N. R., Hemrick-Luecke, S. K., & Clemens, J. A. (1981). Substituted piperazines as central serotonin agonists: Comparative specificity of the post-synatpic actions of quipazine and m-trifluoromethylphenylpiperazine. *Journal of Pharmacology and Experimental Therapeutics, 218,* 636–641.

Fuxe, K., Ogren, S.-O., Agnati, L., Gustafson, J. A., & Jonsson, G. (1977). On the mechanism of action of the antidepressant drugs amitriptyline and nortriptyline. Evidence for 5-hydroxytryptamine receptor blocking activity. *Neuroscience Letters, 6,* 339–343.

Gaddum, J. H., & Picarelli, Z. P. (1957). Two kinds of tryptamine receptor. *British Journal of Pharmacology, 12,* 323–328.

Gerson, S. C., & Baldessarini, R. J. (1980). Motor effects of serotonin in the central nervous system. *Life Sciences, 27,* 1435–1451.

Glennon, R. A. (1986a). Discriminative stimulus properties of the 5-HT$_{1A}$ agonist 8-hydroxy-2-(di-n-propylamino)tetralin (8-OH-DPAT). *Pharmacology, Biochemistry, and Behavior, 25,* 135–139.

Glennon, R. A. (1986b). Discriminative stimulus properties of the serotonergic agent 1-(2,5-dimethoxy-4-iodophenyl)-2-aminopropane (DOI). *Life Sciences, 39,* 825–831.

Glennon, R. A., & Hauck, A. E. (1985). Mechanistic studies on DOM as a discriminative stimulus. *Pharmacology, Biochemistry, and Behavior, 23,* 937–941.

Glennon, R. A., & Lucki, I. (1988). Behavioral models of serotonin receptor activation. In E. Sanders-Bush (Ed.), *The serotonin receptors* (pp. 253–293). Clifton, NJ: Humana.

Glennon, R. A., Pierson, M. E., & McKenney, J. D. (1988). Stimulus generalization of 1-(3-trifluoromethylphenyl)piperazine (TFMPP) to propranolol, pindolol, and mesulergine. *Pharmacology, Biochemistry & Behavior, 29,* 197–199.

Glennon, R. A., Titeler, M., & Young, R. (1984). Evidence for 5-HT₂ involvement in the mechanism of action of hallucinogenic agents. *Life Sciences, 35,* 2502–2511.

Glennon, R. A., Young, R., & Rosecrans, J. A. (1983). Antagonism of the effects of the hallucinogen DOM and the purported 5-HT agonist quipazine by 5-HT₂ antagonists. *European Journal of Pharmacology, 91,* 189–196.

Goldberg, H. L., & Finnerty, R. J. (1979). The comparative efficacy of buspirone and diazepam in the treatment of anxiety. *American Journal of Psychiatry, 136,* 1184–1187.

Goodwin, G. M., De Souza, R. J., & Green, A. R. (1985a). The pharmacology of the hypothermic response in mice to 8-hydroxy-2-(di-n-propylamino)tetralin (8-OH-DPAT). *Neuropharmacology, 24,* 1187–1194.

Goodwin, G. M., De Souza, R. J., & Green, A. R. (1985b). Presynaptic serotonin receptor-mediated response in mice attenuated by antidepressant drugs and electroconvulsive shock. *Nature, 317,* 531–533.

Goodwin, G. M., De Souza, R. J., & Green, A. R. (1986). The effects of a 5-HT₁ receptor ligand isapirone (TVX Q 7821) on 5-HT synthesis and the behavioral effects of 5-HT agonists in mice and rats. *Psychopharmacology, 89,* 382–387.

Goodwin, G. M., De Souza, R. J., Green, A. R., & Heal, D. J. (1987a). The pharmacology of the behavioral and hypothermic responses of rats to 8-hydroxy-2(di-n-propylamino) tetralin (8-OH-DPAT). *Psychopharmacology, 91,* 506–511.

Goodwin, G. M., De Souza, R. J., & Green, A. R. (1987b). Attenuation by electroconvulsive shock and antidepressant drugs of the 5-HT₁ₐ receptor-mediated hypothermia and serotonin syndrome produced by 8-OH-DPAT in the rat. *Psychopharmacology, 91,* 500–505.

Goodwin, G. M., & Green, A. R. (1985). A behavioral and biochemical study in mice and rats of putative selective agonists and antagonists for 5-HT₁ and 5-HT₂ receptors. *British Journal of Pharmacology, 84,* 743–753.

Grahame-Smith, D. G. (1971). Studies in vivo on the relationships between brain tryptophan, brain 5-HT synthesis and hyperactivity in rats treated with a monoamine oxidase inhibitor and L-tryptophan. *Journal of Neurochemistry, 18,* 1053–1066.

Green, A. R., Guy, A. P., & Gardner, C. R. (1984). The behavioral effects of RU 24969, a suggested 5-HT1 receptor agonist in rodents and the effect on the behaviour of treatment with antidepressants. *Neuropharmacology, 23,* 655–661.

Green, A. R., Hall, J. E., & Rees, A. R. (1981). A behavioural and biochemical study in rats of 5-hydroxytryptamine receptor agonists and antagonists, with observations on structure-activity requirements for the agonists. *British Journal of Pharmacology, 73,* 703–719.

Green, R. A., Gillin, J. C., & Wyatt, R. J. (1976). The inhibitory effect of intraventricular administration of serotonin on spontaneous motor activity of rats. *Psychopharmacology, 51,* 81–84.

Gudelsky, G. A., Koenig, J. I., & Meltzer, H. Y. (1986). Thermoregulatory responses to serotonin (5-HT) receptor stimulation in the rat: Evidence for opposing roles of 5-HT₂ and 5-HT₁ₐ receptors. *Neuropharmacology, 25,* 1307–1313.

Haber, B., Gabay, S., Issidorides, M. R., & Alivisatos, S. G. A. (1981). *Serotonin: Current aspects of neurochemistry and function.* New York: Plenum.

Hall, M. D., El Mestikawy, S., Emerit, M. B., Pichat, L., Hamon, M., & Gozlan, H. (1985). [³H]-8-Hydroxy-2-(di-n-propylamino)tetralin binding to pre- and postsynaptic 5-hydroxytryptamine sites in various regions of the rat brain. *Journal of Neurochemistry, 44,* 1685–1696.

Handley, S. L., & Brown, J. (1982). Effects on the 5-hydroxytryptamine-induced head-twitch of drugs with selective actions on alpha1 and alpha2 adrenoceptors. *Neuropharmacology, 21,* 507–510.

Handley, S. L., & Singh, L. (1986a). Neurotransmitters and shaking behaviour—More than a "gut bath" for the brain? *Trends in Pharmacological Sciences, 6,* 324–328.

Handley, S. L., & Singh, L. (1986b). Involvement of the locus coeruleus in the potentiation of the quipazine-induced head-twitch response by diazepam and beta-adrenoceptor agonists. *Neuropharmacology, 25,* 1315–1321.

Heal, D. J., Philpot, J., O'Shaughnessy, K. M., & Davis, J. L. (1986). The influence of central noradrenergic function on 5-HT$_2$ mediated head-twitch responses in mice: Possible implications for the actions of antidepressant drugs. *Psychopharmacology, 89,* 414–420.

Heuring, R. E., & Peroutka, S. J. (1987). Characterization of a novel ^{3}H-5-hydroxytryptamine binding site subtype in bovine brain membranes. *Journal of Neuroscience, 7,* 893–903.

Hjorth, S. (1985). Hypothermia in the rat induced by the potent serotoninergic agent 8-OH-DPAT. *Journal of Neural Transmission, 61,* 131–135.

Hjorth, S., Carlsson, A., Lindberg, P., Sanchez, D., Wilkstrom, H., Arvidsson, L.-E., Hacksell, V., & Nilsson, J. L. G. (1982). 8-Hydroxy-2-(di-n-propylamino)tetralin, 8-OH-DPAT, a potent and selective simplified ergot congener with central 5-HT-receptor stimulating activity. *Journal of Neural Transmission, 55,* 169–188.

Hoyer, D., Engel, G., & Kalkman, H. O. (1985a). Characterization of the 5-HT$_{1B}$ recognition site in rat brain: Binding studies with $(-)$ [^{125}I]iodocyanopindolol. *European Journal of Pharmacology, 118,* 1–12.

Hoyer, D., Engel, G., & Kalkman, H. O. (1985b). Molecular pharmacology of 5-HT$_1$ and 5-HT$_2$ recognition sites in rat and pig brain membranes: Radioligand binding studies with [^{3}H]5-HT, [^{3}H]8-OH-DPAT, $(-)$ [^{125}I]iodocyanopindolol, [^{3}H]mesulergine and [^{3}]ketanserin. *European Journal of Pharmacology, 118,* 13–23.

Hutson, P. H., Donohoe, T. P., & Curzon, G. (1987). Hypothermia induced by the putative 5-HT$_{1A}$ agonists LY165163 and 8-OH-DPAT is not prevented by 5-HT depletion. *European Journal of Pharmacology, 143,* 221–228.

Jacobs, B. L. (1974). Effect of two dopamine receptor blockers on a serotonin-mediated behavioral syndrome in rats. *European Journal of Pharmacology, 27,* 363–366.

Jacobs, B. L. (1976). An animal behavioral model for studying central serotonergic synapses. *Life Sciences, 19,* 777–786.

Jacobs, B. L., & Gelperin, A. (Eds.). (1981). *Serotonin neurotransmission and behavior.* Cambridge, MA: MIT Press.

Jacobs, B. L., & Klemfuss, H. (1975). Brain stem and spinal cord mediation of a serotonergic behavioral syndrome. *Brain Research, 100,* 450–457.

Kennett, G. A., Dourish, C. T., & Curzon, G. (1987). Antidepressant-like action of 5-HT$_{1A}$ agonists and conventional antidepressants in an animal model of depression. *European Journal of Pharmacology, 134,* 265–274.

Lebrecht, V., & Nowack, J. Z. (1980). Effect of single and repeated electoconvulsive shock on serotonergic system in rat brain. II. Behavioral studies. *Neuropharmacology, 19,* 1055–1061.

Leysen, J. E., Niemegeers, C. J. E., Van Nueten, J. M., & Laduron, P. M. (1982). [^{3}H]Ketanserin (R41 468), a selective ^{3}H-ligand for serotonin$_2$ receptor binding sites. *Molecular Pharmacology, 21,* 301–314.

Lorens, S. A. (1978). Some behavioral effects of serotonin depletion depend on method: A comparison of 5,7-dihydroxytryptamine, *p*-chlorophenylalanine, *p*-chloroamphetamine, and electrolytic raphe lesions. *Annals New York Academy of Science, 305,* 532–555.

Lucki, I. (1986). The nonbenzodiazepine anxiolytics buspirone and ipsapirone antagonize serotonin-mediated behavioral responses. *Psychopharmacology, 89,* S55.

Lucki, I. (1988). Rapid discrimination of the stimulus properties of 5-hydroxytryptamine agonists using conditioned taste aversion. *Journal of Pharmacology and Experimental Therapeutics, 247,* 1120–1127.

Lucki, I., Eberle, K. M., & Minugh-Purvis, N. (1987a). The role of the aural head shake reflex in serotonin-mediated head shaking behavior. *Psychopharmacology, 92,* 150–156.

Lucki, I., & Frazer, A. (1982a). Prevention of the serotonin syndrome in rats by repeated administration of monoamine oxidase inhibitors but not tricyclic antidepressants. *Psychopharmacology,* *77,* 205–211.

Lucki, I., & Frazer, A. (1982b). Behavioral effects of indole- and piperazine-type serotonin receptor agonists. *Society for Neuroscience Abstracts, 8,* 101.

Lucki, I., & Frazer, A. (1985). Changes in behavior associated with serotonin receptors following repeated treatment of rats with antidepressant drugs: In L. S. Seiden & R. L. Balster (Eds.), *Behavioral pharmacology: Current status* (pp. 339–357). New York: Alan Liss.

Lucki, I., & Harvey, J. A. (1979). Increased sensitivity to d- and l-amphetamine action after midbrain raphe lesions as measured by locomotor activity. *Neuropharmacology, 18,* 243–249.

Lucki, I., & Minugh-Purvis, N. (1987). Serotonin-induced head shaking behavior in rats does not involve receptors located in the frontal cortex. *Brain Research, 420,* 403–406.

Lucki, I., Nobler, M. S., & Frazer, A. (1984). Differential actions of serotonin antagonists on two behavioral models of serotonin receptor activation in the rat. *Journal of Pharmacology and Experimental Therapeutics, 228,* 133–139.

Lucki, I., Sills, M. A., Frazer, A., & Nelson, D. L. (1987b). Pyridyl indole agonists and serotonin (5-HT) receptor subtypes and behavior. *Federation Proceedings, 46,* 965.

Lucki, I., Ward, H. R., & Frazer, A. (1989). The effect of 1-(m-chlorophenyl)piperazine (m-CPP) and 1-(m-trifluoromethylphenyl)piperazine (TFMPP) on locomotor activity. *Journal of Pharmacology and Experimental Therapeutics,* in press.

Maj, J., Palider, W., & Rawlow, A. (1979). Trazadone, a central serotonin antagonist and agonist. *Journal of Neural Transmission, 44,* 237–248.

Mansbach, R. S., & Barrett, J. E. (1987). Discriminative stimulus properties of buspirone in the pigeon. *Journal of Pharmacology and Experimental Therapeutics, 240,* 364–369.

Marcinkiewicz, M., Verge, D., Gozlan, H., Pichat, L., & Hamon, M. (1984). Autoradiographic evidence for the heterogeneity of 5-HT$_1$ sites in the rat brain. *Brain Research, 291,* 159–163.

Matthews, W. D., & Smith, C. D. (1980). Pharmacological profile of a model for central serotonin receptor activation. *Life Sciences, 26,* 1397–1403.

McKenney, J. D., & Glennon, R. A. (1986). TFMPP may produce its stimulus effects via a 5-HT$_{1B}$ mechanism. *Pharmacology, Biochemistry, and Behavior, 24,* 43–47.

Mendelson, S. D., & Gorzalka, B. B. (1988). Differential roles of 5-HT receptor subtypes in female sexual behavior. In T. Archer, P. Bevan, & L. Cools (Eds.), *Behavioral pharmacology of serotonin.* Hillsdale, NJ: Lawrence Erlbaum Associates.

Mendelson, S. D., & Gorzalka, B. B. (1989). 5-HT$_{1A}$ receptors: Differential involvement in female and male sexual behavior in the rat. *Physiology and Behavior, 37,* 345–351.

Middlemiss, D. N., & Fozard, J. R. (1983). 8-Hydroxy-2-(di-n-propylamino)tetralin discriminates between subtypes of the 5-HT1 recognition site. *European Journal of Pharmacology, 90,* 151–153.

Modigh, K. (1972). Central and peripheral effects of 5-hydroxytryptophan on motor activity in mice. *Psychopharmacologia, 88,* 445–450.

Nahorski, S. R., & Willcocks, A. L. (1983). Interactions of beta-adrenoceptor antagonists with 5-hydroxytryptamine receptor subtypes in rat cerebral cortex. *British Journal of Pharmacology, 78,* 107P.

Neale, R. F., Fallon, S. L., Boyar, W. C., Wasley, J. W. F., Martin, L. L., Stone, G. A., Glaeser, B. S., Sinton, C. M., & Williams, M. (1987). Biochemical and pharmacological characterization of CGS 12066B, a selective serotonin-1B agonist. *European Journal of Pharmacology, 136,* 1–9.

Niemegeers, C. J. E., Colpaert, F. C., Leysen, J. E., Awouters, F., & Janssen, P. A. J. (1983). Mescaline-induced head twitches in the rat: An in vivo method to evaluate serotonin S2 antagonists. *Drug Development Research, 3,* 123–135.

Offord, S. J., DeAngelo, T. M., Wang, H. L., & Frazer, A. (1987). Comparison of the affinity of serotonin agonists for th 5-HT-1A receptor with their potency at eliciting a 5-HT-1A receptor-mediated response. *Society for Neuroscience Abstracts, 13,* 343.

Offord, S. J., Ordway, G. A., & Frazer, A. (1988). Application of [^{125}I]iodocyanopindolol to measure 5-hydroxytryptamine$_{1B}$ receptors in the brain of the rat. *Journal of Pharmacology and Experimental Therapeutics, 244,* 144–153.

Ogren, S. O., Fuxe, K., Agnati, L. F., Gustafsson, J. A., Jonsson, G., & Holm, A. C. (1979). Reevaluation of the indoleamine hypothesis of depression. Evidence for a reduction of functional activity of central 5-HT systems by antidepressant drugs. *Journal of Neural Transmission, 46,* 85–103.

Oksenberg, D., & Peroutka, S. J. (1988). Antagonism of 5-hydroxytryptamine$_{1A}$ (5-HT$_{1A}$) receptor-mediated modulation of adenylate cyclase activity by pindolol and propranolol isomers. *Biochemical Pharmacology, 37,* 3429–3433.

Osborne, N. N. (Ed.). (1982). *Biology of serotonergic transmission.* New York: Wiley.

Overton, D. A. (1987). Applications and limitations of the drug discrimination method for the study of drug abuse. In M. A. Bozarth (Ed.), *Methods of assessing the reinforcing properties of abused drugs* (pp. 291–340). New York: Springer-Verlag.

Pazos, A., Cortes, R., & Palacios, J. M. (1985). Quantitative autoradiographic mapping of serotonin receptors in the rat brain. II. Serotonin-2 receptors. *Brain Research, 346,* 231–249.

Pazos, A., Hoyer, D., & Palacios, J. M. (1984). The binding of serotonergic ligands to the porcine choroid plexus: Characterization of a new type of serotonin recognition site. *European Journal of Pharmacology, 106,* 539–546.

Pedigo, N. W., Yamamura, H. I., & Nelson, D. L. (1981). Discrimination of multiple ^{3}H-5-hydroxytryptamine binding sites by the neuroleptic spiperone in rat brain. *Journal of Neurochemistry, 36,* 220–226.

Peroutka, S. J. (1986). Pharmacological differentiation and characterization of 5-HT1A, 5-HT1B, and 5-HT1C binding sites in rat frontal cortex. *Journal of Neurochemistry, 47,* 529–540.

Peroutka, S. J., Lebovitz, R. M., & Snyder, S. H. (1981). Two distinct central serotonin receptors with different physiological functions. *Science, 212,* 827–829.

Peroutka, S. J., & Snyder, S. H. (1979). Multiple serotonin receptors: Differential binding of [3H]-5-hydroxytryptamine, [3H]-lysergic acid diethylamide and [3H]-spiroperidol. *Molecular Pharmacology, 16,* 687–699.

Peroutka, S. J., & Snyder, S. H. (1980). Long-term antidepressant treatment decreases spiroperidol-labelled serotonin receptor binding. *Science, 210,* 88–90.

Samanin, R., Mennini, T., Ferraris, A., Bendotti, C., Borsini, F., & Garattini, S. (1979). m-Chlorophenylpiperazine: A central serotonin agonist causing powerful anorexia in rats. *Naunyn Schmiedeberg's Archives of Pharmacology, 308,* 159–163.

Schechter, L. E., & Simansky, K. J. (1988). 1-(2,5-Dimethoxy-4-iodophenyl)-2-aminopropane (DOI) exerts an anorexic action that is blocked by 5-HT$_2$ antagonists in rats. *Psychopharmacology, 94,* 342–346.

Schlosberg, A. J., & Harvey, J. A. (1979). Effects of L-Dopa and L-5-hydroxytryptophan on locomotor activity of the rat after selective or combined destruction of central catecholamine and serotonin neurons. *Journal of Pharmacology and Experimental Therapeutics, 211,* 296–304.

Schuster, C. R., Fischman, M. W., & Johanson, C. E. (1981). Internal stimulus control and subjective effects of drugs. In T. Thompson & C. E. Johanson (Eds.), *Behavioral pharmacology of human drug dependence* (pp. 116–129). Washington, D.C.: NIDA Research Monograph 37.

Sills, M. A., Lucki, I., & Frazer, A. (1985). Development of selective tolerance to the serotonin behavioral syndrome and suppression of locomotor activity after repeated administration of either 5-MeODMT or mCPP. *Life Sciences, 36,* 2463–2469.

Sills, M. A., Wolfe, B. B., & Frazer, A. (1984). Determination of selective and non-selective compounds for the 5-HT1A and 5-HT1B receptor subtypes in rat frontal cortex. *Journal of Pharmacology and Experimental Therapeutics, 231,* 480–487.

Sloviter, R. S., Drust, E. G., & Conner, J. D. (1978a). Specificity of a rat behavioral model for serotonin receptor activation. *Journal of Pharmacology and Experimental Therapeutics, 206,* 339–347.

148 LUCKI

Sloviter, R. S., Drust, E. G., & Conner, J. D. (1978b). Evidence that serotonin mediates some behavioral effects of amphetamine. *Journal of Pharmacology and Experimental Therapeutics, 206*, 348–352.

Sloviter, R. S., Drust, E. G., Damiano, B. P., & Conner, J. D. (1980). A common mechanism for lysergic acid, indole alkylamine and phenethylamine hallucinogens: Serotonergic mediation of behavioral effects in rats. *Journal of Pharmacology and Experimental Therapeutics, 214*, 231–238.

Smith, L. M., & Peroutka, S. J. (1986). Differential effects of 5-hydroxytryptamine1A selective drugs on the 5-HT behavioral syndrome. *Pharmacology, Biochemistry and Behavior, 24*, 1513–1519.

Spencer Jr., D. G., & Traber, J. (1987). The interoceptive discriminative stimuli induced by the novel putative anxiolytic TVX Q 7821: behavioral evidence for the specific involvement of serotonin 5-HT$_{1A}$ receptors. *Psychopharmacology, 91*, 25–29.

Sprouse, J. S., & Aghajanian, G. K. (1987). Electrophysiological responses of serotoninergic dorsal raphe neurons to 5-HT$_{1A}$ and 5-HT$_{1B}$ agonists. *Synapse, 1*, 3–9.

Svensson, L., & Ahlenius, S. (1983). Enhancement by putative 5-HT receptor agonist 8-OH-2-(di-n-propylamino)tetralin of the acoustic startle response in the rat. *Psychopharmacology, 79*, 104–107.

Titeler, M., Lyon, R. A., & Glennon, R. A. (1988). Radioligand binding evidence implicates the brain 5-HT$_2$ receptor as a site of action for LSD and phenylisopropylamine hallucinogens. *Psychopharmacology, 94*, 213–216.

Tondo, L., Conway, P. G., & Brunswick, D. J. (1985). Labeling *in vivo* of *beta*-adrenergic receptors in the central nervous system of the rat after administration of [^{125}I]iodopindolol. *Journal of Pharmacology and Experimental Therapeutics, 235*, 1–9.

Tricklebank, M. D., Forler, C., & Fozard, J. R. (1985). The involvement of subtypes of the 5-HT1 receptor and of catecholaminergic systems in the behavioural response to 8-hydroxy-2-(di-n-propylamino)tetralin in the rat. *European Journal of Pharmacology, 106*, 271–282.

Tricklebank, M. D., Middlemiss, D. N., & Neill, J. (1986). Pharmacological analysis of the behavioural and thermoregulatory effects of the putative 5-HT1 receptor agonist, RU 24969, in the rat. *Neuropharmacology, 25*, 877–886.

Tricklebank, M. D., Neill, J., Kidd, E. J., & Fozard, J. R. (1987). Mediation of the discriminative stimulus properties of 8-hydroxy-2-(di-n-propylamino) tetralin (8-OH DPAT) by the putative 5-HT$_{1A}$ receptor. *European Journal of Pharmacology, 133*, 47–56.

Trulson, M. E., & Jacobs, B. L. (1976). Behavioral evidence for the rapid release of CNS serotonin by PCA and fenfluramine. *European Journal of Pharmacology, 36*, 149–154.

Vetulani, J., Bednarczyk, B., Reichenberg, K., & Rokosz, A. (1980). Head twitches induced by LSD and quipazine: Similarities and differences. *Neuropharmacology, 19*, 155–158.

Vetulani, J., Lebrecht, U., & Pilc, A. (1981). Enhancement of responsiveness of the central serotonergic system and serotonin-2 receptor density in rat frontal cortex by electroconvulsive treatment. *European Journal of Pharmacology, 76*, 81–85.

Warbritton III, J. D., Stewart, R. M., & Baldessarini, R. J. (1978). Decreased locomotor activity and attenuation of amphetamine hyperactivity with intraventricular infusion of serotonin in the rat. *Brain Research, 143*, 373–382.

6 Nutritional Aspects of Drug Action on Behavior

Kathleen M. Kantak
Boston University

INTRODUCTION

The study of the effects of drugs upon behavior began over 30 years ago. The field of Behavioral Pharmacology grew with the basic assumptions that because drugs change neurochemical functioning in the brain, they are capable of altering a variety of behaviors. The past 3 decades have been rich in describing the psychoactive properties of drugs. The findings that dietary nutrients can also change brain neurochemical functions have given rise not only to the study of relationships between diet and behavior, but also to the effects of nutrients on drug interactions with behavior. These latter aspects have been termed Dietary Behavioral Pharmacology (Dews, 1986). Much of this literature has mainly focused on manipulations of protein, carbohydrates, and individual amino acids. Other nutrients are also capable of interactions with the brain. Most notable are reports of certain vitamins and minerals having a modulatory effect on behavior and drug action.

Until recently, most scientists did not take the anecdotal evidence of acute behavioral effects of diet seriously because such effects were considered too implausible (Dews, 1986). Consider for the moment some titles of articles that have appeared during the past few years: "Scientists Ponder Diet's Behavioral Effects" (Simmons, 1985); "Diet And Human Behavior: How Much Do They Affect Each Other?" (Kruesi, 1986); "Behavioral Changes Caused by Nutrients" (Lieberman, 1986). Such considerations and reflections have arisen because of the increased scientific rigor that has been applied to this field of research. Dietary Behavioral Pharmacology has emerged as a legitimate field of study. It is the purpose of this review to capture the spirit of this rigor by focusing information on three nutrients: the amino acid tryptophan, the mineral magnesium, and the vitamin ascorbic acid (vitamin C). Recent information on how these nutrients interact with drugs makes these nutrients of special interest to Behavioral Pharmacology.

TRYPTOPHAN

Tryptophan Neurochemistry

Tryptophan, an essential amino acid, is the precursor to serotonin (5-hydroxytryptamine, 5-HT). The initial step is the hydroxylation of L-tryptophan by tryptophan hydroxylase to L-5-hydroxytryptophan (Udenfriend, Titus, Weissbach, & Peterson, 1956; Udenfriend & Weissback, 1958). L-5-hydroxytryptophan is then decarboxylated to 5-HT by L-aromatic amino acid decarboxylase. Because tryptophan is an essential amino acid, the consumption of food has a powerful influence over tryptophan availability and 5-HT metabolism in the central nervous system. Tryptophan is present in two forms in the blood; that which is bound to albumin and that which is free (McMenamy & Oncly, 1958). The free tryptophan is the only form that can cross the blood brain barrier to enter the brain. Because of this unique feature for tryptophan binding to albumin, there is, under normal conditions less free tryptophan (10%) than there is bound tryptophan (90%). In addition, tryptophan competes with five other neutral amino acids (phenylalanine, tyrosine, leucine, isoleucine, and valine) for transport into the brain from the blood (Blasberg & Lajtha, 1965). The amino acid that has the highest ratio of the concentration of itself to the sum of the concentrations of all the others is preferentially taken up into the brain. With little free tryptophan available to enter the brain, the tryptophan hydroxylase enzyme is normally unsaturated (Carlsson et al., 1972; Colmenares, Wurtman, & Fernstrom, 1975). The K_m for tryptophan hydroxylase in rat brain is 50 uM and since the concentration of tryptophan is also approximately 50 uM, this enzyme is 50% saturated (Kaufman, 1974). Thus, treatments that decrease tryptophan availability to the brain (tryptophan-free diet, protein consumption) decrease central 5-HT metabolism and treatments which increase tryptophan availability to the brain (tryptophan load, carbohydrate consumption, food deprivation) increase central 5-HT metabolism (Curzon, Joseph, & Knott, 1972; Fernstrom & Hirsch, 1975; Fernstrom & Jacoby, 1975; Fernstrom & Wurtman, 1971; Gibbons et al., 1979; Kantak, Wayner, & Stein, 1978).

Behavioral Effects of Tryptophan Modulation

The modulation of tryptophan levels has been shown to produce some behavioral changes that are consistent with drug manipulations on the serotonergic system. Maintaining rats on a tryptophan-free diet for 4 to 6 days induces predatory mouse killing in nonkiller rats and facilitates this muricide response in killer rats (Gibbons et al., 1979). However, supplementing the tryptophan-free diet with tryptophan loads (0.5% or 2%) does not produce any behavioral changes different from control although brain 5-HT and 5-HIAA are increased. In defensively aggressive rats, a tryptophan-free diet produces increases in shock-induced fighting and muricide (Kantak, Hegstrand, Whitman, & Eichelman, 1980a). A 5% load of tryptophan fails to alter these behaviors. In contrast to defensive and predatory behaviors, offensive aggressive behavior in isolated mice is reduced by a tryptophan deficient diet (Kantak, Hegstrand, & Eichelman, 1980b). A 5% tryptophan load fails to influence this behavior as well. In general, behavioral reactivity to stimuli is enhanced by a dietary tryptophan deficiency. This includes sensitivity to pain (Messing, Fisher, Phebus, & Lytle, 1976) and acoustic startle response (Walters, Davis, & Sheard, 1979) in addition to defensive and predatory aggression. Tryptophan loads alone usually produce no changes in aggression and other behaviors such as motor activity (Grahame-Smith, 1971), pain sensitivity (Hole & Marsden, 1975), sexual behavior (Tagliamonte, Tagliamonte, Perez-Cruet, & Gessa, 1972), and feeding behavior (Weinberger, Knapp, & Mandell, 1978) which typically change in response to drugs which enhance central 5-HT activity.

In humans, alterations in 5-HT are thought to be associated with aggression, sleep disturbances, and depression. One important study concerned biogenic amine metabolites in the CSF of a group of military men with no history of major psychiatric illness, but with various personality disorders (Brown, Goodwin, Bellenger, & Goyer, 1981). Scored histories of aggressive behavior show a significant negative correlation with CSF 5-HIAA. Those with histories of suicide attempts show similar findings (Brown et al., 1982). In schizophrenic patients who exhibit impulsive aggression, tryptophan (4 or 8 gm per day) has been shown to produce a 30% decrease in physical assault, verbal abuse and uncontrolled behavior as measured on a word checklist (Morand, Young, & Ervin, 1983). Following acute lowering of tryptophan by feeding a balanced mixture of amino acids devoid of tryptophan to normal volunteers, no effects on experimentally-induced aggression or on a checklist score for hostility are found (Young, 1986). This is an interesting contrast between the chronic effect of tryptophan administration in mentally disturbed patients and the effects of acute tryptophan depletion in mentally normal subjects.

Hartman & Greenwald (1984) studied the effects of 1,2,3,4,5,10, and 15 gm L-tryptophan and placebo, each given once in a crossover design to subjects 21–35 years-of-age. Sleep-onset latencies were reduced from a placebo mean of 24.2 min to means ranging from 10.8 to 16.1 min after L-tryptophan administration. These findings are similar to those reported earlier by Griffiths, Lester, & Coulter (1972). The results of these studies indicate that L-tryptophan may reduce the time required for sleep onset when baseline latencies are longer than normal (a normal latency is approximately 15 min). In situations not conducive to sleep and/or in subjects with short sleep latencies, L-tryptophan does not significantly reduce sleep onset time (Spinweber, Ursin, Hilbert, & Hilderbrand, 1983).

The use of tryptophan in depression has received considerable attention, largely owing to the facts that there are lower than normal concentrations of 5-HIAA in the CSF of depressed patients than in normal controls or recovered depressed patients (Ashcroft et al., 1966). It is estimated that 30% of depressed patients can be classified into a subgroup that is marked by suicidal tendencies and correlated with lower 5-HT turnover (Traskman, Asberg, Bertilsson, & Sjostrand, 1981). In some cases, tryptophan alone is as effective as electroconvulsive therapy (Coppen, Shaw, Herzberg, & Maggs, 1967), and amitriptyline (Herrington, Bruce, Johnston, & Lader, 1976) in the treatment of depression. In many studies tryptophan alone appears to be largely ineffective (Cooper & Datta, 1980; Murphy et al., 1974).

Interactions with Tryptophan and Drugs

It was previously indicated that excess tryptophan alone in both intact animals and normal humans does not have as robust an effect upon behavior as tryptophan deficiencies do. This may be related to the ability of the serotonergic system under normal conditions to intraneuronally metabolize the excess tryptophan without the serotonin becoming functionally active, i.e., released and available to the post-synaptic receptor (Grahame-Smith, 1971). When excess tryptophan is administered in conjunction with other drugs, the behavioral altering properties of excess tryptophan become more apparent.

In a study on aggressive behavior in rats, 5,7-dihydroxytryptamine (5,7-DHT) and septal lesions were used to enhance shock-induced fighting and mouse-killing (Kantak, Hegstrand, & Eichelman, 1981). Following lesioning, it was determined if a 5% tryptophan-loaded diet could reverse the lesion effects. Results indicate that shock-induced fighting could be maintained at normal levels following dietary tryptophan loading in 5,7-DHT lesioned rats and septally lesioned rats (Fig. 6.1). Mouse-killing was not significantly elevated by the concentration of 5,7-DHT used in this study. Following septal lesions, dietary tryptophan loads could not reverse the increase in mouse-killing behavior. Depletions of 5-HT and 5-HIAA following 5,7-DHT were distributed throughout the brain; whereas the depletions following septal lesions were confined to the hippocampus among the brain regions examined (hippocampus, forebrain, rest of brain). Small repletions of 5-HT and 5-HIAA following tryptophan loading in septally lesioned rats were confined to the hippocampus as well, while repletions were globally measured in 5,7-DHT lesioned rats. Because of the striking similarities in some of the behavioral changes following the two independent, dissimilar lesioning procedures, serotonergic mechanisms within the hippocampus

SHOCK — INDUCED FIGHTING

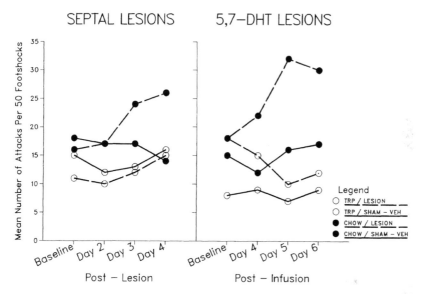

FIG. 6.1. Mean number of attacks per 50 footshocks in septal lesion experiment (left) and 5,7-DHT lesion experiment (right). Data were recorded during Baseline and days 2–4 Post Septal Lesion and during Baseline and days 4–6 Post 5,7-DHT Infusion. Taken from Kantak et al. (1981).

may be critical for the behavioral reversal in shock-induced fighting. Others (Gibbons et al., 1980) have indicated that a reduction in serotonergic activity within the septum is of primary importance for maintaining mouse-killing. If septal, this could account for the lack of a reversal in mouse-killing in tryptophan-loaded, septally lesioned rats since electrolytic lesioning would destroy the neuronal elements in this area which probably would prevent the synthesis of 5-HT from excess tryptophan.

An interaction of tryptophan and para-chlorophenylalanine (PCPA) on sleep behavior in rats has also been reported (Borbely, Neuhaus, & Tobler, 1981). Initially. PCPA causes slow wave sleep to increase and REM sleep to decrease. Following 1 to 2 days of insomnia, both slow wave sleep and REM sleep are depressed at a time when 5-HT is depleted. Tryptophan (150 mg/kg) 28 hr after PCPA causes an increase in brain 5-HT and temporarily increases slow wave sleep and REM sleep. This is thought to be related to the fact that during sleep, there is reduced raphe activity. Tryptophan in PCPA pretreated rats depresses raphe firing rate and thus produces an enhancement in sleep (Gallager & Aghajanian, 1976).

Perhaps one of the more interesting interactions between tryptophan and drugs in animals is the one between tryptophan and d-amphetamine self-administration. Lyness (1983) demonstrated that increasing doses of tryptophan (25, 50 and 100 mg/kg) reduce responding for d-amphetamine in a time-dependent manner. These effects are not due to sedation since tryptophan treated rats do maintain behavior on a FR40 food reinforcement schedule. Tryptophan did not alter DA, DOPAC or HVA in the nucleus accumbens, a brain site related to the reinforcing action of stimulants (Wise, 1984). Peripheral injections of tryptophan did increase brain levels of tryptophan, 5-HT and 5-HIAA with a time course similar to the attenuation of self-administration rates. This indicates that a 5-HT rather than DA effect may be causative in the decrease in self-administration rate. It was further demonstrated that 5,7-DHT pretreatment enhances d-amphetamine self-administration; whereas, fluoxetine, quipazine, and tryptophan pretreatment decrease the self-administration of d-amphetamine (Leccese & Lyness, 1984). 5-HT antagonists cyproheptadine and methysergide potentiate the 5,7-DHT effect.

This attenuation of d-amphetamine self-administration by tryptophan raises the interesting question: ''Is tryptophan a substitute for d-amphetamine, having reward or positive reinforcing properties as other substitutes for d-amphetamine have?'' Although the self-administration of tryptophan following the self-administration of d-amphetamine has not been examined, there is evidence that tryptophan does not affect conditioned place preference and is therefore not in itself reinforcing (Smith et al., 1986). One would not expect, therefore, that tryptophan acts as a substitute for d-amphetamine. In spite of a lack of a clear understanding of the mechanism for this interaction, the potential use of tryptophan in the treatment of stimulant abuse is compelling, especially since tryptophan can decrease d-amphetamine self-administration without producing tolerance (Smith et al., 1986).

Although the use of tryptophan alone has been largely ineffective in the treatment of human depression, tryptophan may be best employed as an antidepressant potentiator. In combination with MAO inhibitors and tricyclic antidepressants, tryptophan has been shown to be superior over treatment with the drug alone (Coppen, Shaw, & Farrell, 1963; Pare, 1963). There are several reasons why tryptophan fails to be effective (Chouinard, Young, Annable, & Sourkes, 1979). There appears to be a therapeutic window for tryptophan efficacy which is approximately 6 gm/day. Also high tryptophan doses induce the liver enzyme tryptophan pyrolase which can shunt tryptophan away from the brain. Inclusion of a tryptophan pyrolase inhibitor, such as nicotinamide, has proven to be beneficial in increasing the effectiveness of tryptophan for depression. Lastly, there may be only a subgroup who benefit with tryptophan, because 5-HT dysfunction may be the cause of depression in only some individuals (Moller, Kirk, & Fremming, 1976).

Summary

A central finding that emerges from the review of the above studies is that tryptophan alone does not have robust effects in intact animals and normal humans. In some cases in humans, tryptophan alone is effective; this occurs in aggressive schizophrenic patients, individuals with long sleep latencies and individuals with major depression. These studies imply that when brain function is not normal, tryptophan can be effective to bring about a behavioral change. This idea is supported by the animal literature as well. Perhaps the most important benefits of tryptophan are when it is used in conjunction with other drugs to enhance their effectiveness (such as with anti-depressants) or to reduce their effectiveness (such as with stimulant use). This also implies that tryptophan is effective when the brain is functioning differently than usual because of the presence of drugs.

MAGNESIUM

Magnesium Neurochemistry

Magnesium (Mg^{2+}) is the fourth most abundant mineral in the brain with an important regulatory role in cellular membrane function (Aikawa, 1971). It is inhibitory to nerve cell conductance and opposes the actions of calcium on neurotransmitter release. In addition, Mg^{2+} is an important cofactor in activating tryptophan hydroxylase (Boadle-Biber, 1978) and tyrosine hydroxylase (Raese et al., 1979). Mg^{2+} is necessary for binding of the neurotransmitter on the serotonin receptor (Nelson et al., 1980), dopamine receptor (Usdin, Creese, & Snyder, 1980), beta-adrenergic receptor (Lefkowitz, Mullikin, & Caron, 1976), alpha-adrenergic receptor (Rouot, U'Pritchard, & Snyder, 1980), and the opiate receptor (Pasternak, Snowman, & Snyder, 1975). Mg^{2+} activates adenylate cyclase (Kanoff, Hegstrand, & Greengard, 1977) and phosphodiesterase (Kakiuchi, Yamazuki, & Teshima, 1972). Thus, these *in vitro* studies demonstrate that Mg^{2+} is important for pre- and postsynaptic neurotransmitter functioning.

Restriction to 6%–9% of the Mg^{2+} requirement for 10 days fails to alter regional levels of 5-HT, DA and NE (Chutkow & Tyce, 1979). However, after 16 days on a low Mg^{2+} diet, regional levels of 5-HT are reduced (Essman, 1980), revealing possible time related reductions in brain biogenic amines with Mg^{2+} deficiency. There is also evidence for a reduction in the affinity of membrane bound alpha- and beta-adrenergic receptors with decreasing Mg^{2+} concentration (Glossmann, Hornung, & Presek, 1980; Williams, Mullikin, & Lefkowitz, 1978).

Dopamine binding studies have demonstrated that divalent cations, including Mg^{2+}, Li^{2+}, Ca^{2+} and Mn^{2+}, increase the B_{max} associated with ^3H-spiroperidol binding in rat striata (Usdin et al., 1980). Mg^{2+} produces a maximum increase of 200% above the control, although Mn^{2+} is the most potent cation. It was determined that divalent cations do not actually increase the number of receptors, but prevent the time-dependent degradation of ligand binding to the receptor. More recent studies demonstrate that Mg^{2+} allows for high affinity binding of dopamine to the D-2 antagonist preferring receptor in rat striatal membranes (DeVries & Beart, 1985; Hamblin & Creese, 1982). In fact, Mg^{2+} is capable of potently enhancing dopamine affinity on D-2 receptors by a factor of 1000 (a micromolar to nanomolar potency change). Furthermore, Mg^{2+} decreases the affinity of dopamine antagonists at the D-2 receptor (Wantanabe, George, & Seeman, 1985). Thus, because of the ability of Mg^{2+} to alter neurotransmitter functions, it is also likely to produce effects that also alter behavior.

Behavioral Effects of Magnesium Modulation

The effects of Mg^{2+} alterations on behavior are as diverse as those of tryptophan. Intraventricular injections of 20 umoles Mg^{2+} elicit an eating response approximately three to four times greater than normal in sheep (Seoane, Cote, & Liretto, 1981). Similar effects are observed with Ca^{2+}. Coadministration of 10 umoles Mg^{2+} and 10 umoles Ca^{2+} do not antagonize each other, but instead elicits an eating response that is additive and equal to that elicited by 20 umoles of Ca^{2+}.

Chronically elevating plasma Mg^{2+} improves hippocampal frequency potentiation and reversal learning in aged and young rats (Landfield & Morgan, 1984). Elevating the extracellular Mg^{2+}/Ca^{2+} ratio in a bathing medium had been the only procedure yet reported that specifically improved brain frequency potentiation (or paired-pulse facilitation), in the absence of general excitability increases. In the reversal learning study, 25-month-old rats and 9-month-old rats were tested on a reversal learning task in a T-maze to avoid shock. Old rats on high Mg^{2+} diets and both young groups (high Mg^{2+} diet and control diet) not only make more correct choices on retention trials, but also run the maze more quickly. On reversal acquisition trials, there are no differences among groups, although high Mg^{2+} groups tended to perform better than controls.

Extensive studies on Mg^{2+} modulation and aggression have been conducted. There are concentration-dependent and time-dependent reductions in offensive aggressive behavior in mice with Mg^{2+} deficiencies that do not appear to be related to debilitation of the animals (Kantak, 1988). Defensive behavior is affected in the opposite manner as offensive behavior. This helps to establish the lack of nonspecific behavioral suppressant effects of low Mg^{2+} treatment. The changes in aggression are accompanied by concentration-dependent and time-dependent reductions in functional DA and NE activity, as measured by a reduced behavioral response to 2 mg/kg apomorphine and 1.5 mg/kg l-amphetamine, respectively. These latter data support the *in vitro* evidence that suggest low magnesium reduces the production and utilization of catecholamines. Mg^{2+} excess studies indicate that low doses of $MgCl_2$ (15 and 30 mg/kg) enhance and high doses of $MgCl_2$ (125 and 250 mg/kg) suppress offensive aggression in mice (Izenwasser, Garcia-Valdez, & Kantak, 1986). Taken together with the deficiency studies, an interesting relationship between level of magnesium and level of offensive aggression emerges where deficiencies and high excess inhibit these behaviors and moderate excesses facilitate these behaviors. This is a classical inverted—U shape function (Fig. 6.2). In addition, behavioral tolerance develops to the aggression enhancing effects of $MgCl_2$ (Izenwasser et al., 1986). Increasing doses of $MgCl_2$ also increase DA and NE functions as evidenced by shifts to the left in the dose responses to apomorphine and l-amphetamine (Kantak & Adlerstein, 1985). The fact that Mg^{2+} produces an inverted—U shape function toward offensive aggression, produces tolerance at behavioral activating doses, and has activating effects on catecholamine systems, are highly suggestive that Mg^{2+} has stimulant-like properties. The fact

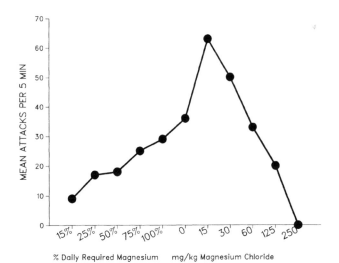

% Daily Required Magnesium   mg/kg Magnesium Chloride

FIG. 6.2. Composite graph of the mean attacks per 5 min in male resident mice following diets containing various percents (15, 25, 50, 75 and 100%) of the daily required magnesium (deficiency) and injection of various doses (0, 15, 30, 60, 125 and 250 mg/kg) of magnesium chloride (excess). The diets were fed for 3 weeks prior to testing and subcutaneous injections were made 5 min before testing. Derived from data described in Izenwasser et al. (1986) and Kantak (1988).

that Mg^{2+} also enhances performance on a learning task supports this notion (Landfield & Morgan, 1984).

Some autistic children respond favorably to high doses of vitamin B_6 and Mg^{2+}. In an early study (LeLord, Callaway, & Muh, 1982) Mg^{2+} was included with this treatment because large doses of B_6 can cause irritability (defensiveness) and hypersensitivity to sound and light. Fifteen out of 44 children showed moderate clinical improvement with worsening on termination of the treatment. Reinstitution of the B_6/Mg^{2+} treatment resulted in improvement again. The improvement with this treatment corresponded to a decrease in urinary HVA levels to the levels found in control children. Others have demonstrated that B_6 plus Mg^{2+} works better than B_6 alone or Mg^{2+} alone (Barthelemy et al., 1981; Martineau, Barthelemy, Garreau, & LeLord, 1985). Small doses of Mg^{2+} (10—15 mg/kg/day) are sufficient to bring about a clinical improvement rating as well as reduce urinary HVA levels when given in conjunction with B_6. It is not clear if this combination is successful because of their action as nutrients or their influence on neurotransmitter metabolism.

Interactions with Magnesium and Drugs

As indicated above, Mg^{2+} may have stimulant-like properties. If so, then one prediction would be that Mg^{2+} would interact with stimulant drugs, such as cocaine, and alter their potency. In a study testing this prediction (Fig. 6.3), the acute administration of cocaine produced an inverted—U shape function on offensive mouse aggression in a normal Mg^{2+} control group and a 30 mg/kg $MgCl_2$ excess group (Kantak, 1986). However, there was a shift to the left in the dose response to cocaine in the excess group. The average dose of cocaine that produced the maximum facilitation in attacks was 0.53 mg/kg in the excess group and 10.0 mg/kg in the control group; this is an increase in cocaine potency by almost a factor of 20 with excess Mg^{2+}. Conversely, a Mg^{2+} deficient diet (15% of daily requirement) reduces the potency of cocaine. In fact, no facilitation in aggression could be detected up to a dose of 40 mg/kg cocaine. The chronic administration (15 days) of 0.5 mg/kg cocaine produces reductions in offensive aggression (Kantak, 1986). Low doses (15 and 30 mg/kg) of $MgCl_2$ and a Mg^{2+} deficient diet maintain this inhibitory effect. The most interesting finding from this study, however, was the prevention of a reduction in aggression in mice who were injected with 125 mg/kg $MgCl_2$ following chronic cocaine. This indicates that a high dose of $MgCl_2$ is preventing the disruptive effect of chronic cocaine, perhaps by maintaining catecholamine activity which is normally reduced by chronic cocaine (Dackis & Gold, 1984).

It is clear from the acute study that excess Mg^{2+} increases the potency of cocaine, and low Mg^{2+} decreases the potency of cocaine. The fact that excess Mg^{2+} could increase the potency of cocaine is consistent with *in vitro* studies showing that dopamine agonist action is facilitated by Mg^{2+} and other divalent

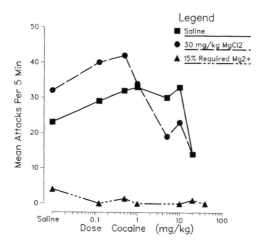

FIG. 6.3. Mean attacks per 5 min in male resident mice following various doses (0, .1, .5, 1, 5, 10, 20 and 40 mg/kg) cocaine HCl and pretreatment with either saline (control), 30 mg/kg magnesium chloride (excess) or a 15% required magnesium diet (deficiency). Injections were made 5 min before testing and the diet was fed for 3 weeks prior to testing. Drawn from data described in Kantak (1986).

cations. Theoretically, the behavioral potency of dopamine antagonist action should be reduced by $MgCl_2$ excess and enhanced by a Mg^{2+} deficiency. As predicted (Fig. 6.4), the acute administration of haloperidol produces dose dependent decreases in offensive aggression with the dose response in the excess group shifted to the right of the control group and the dose response in the deficient group shifted to the left of the control group (Kantak, unpublished findings). The chronic administration (15 days) of 0.5 mg/kg haloperidol produces the same effects as chronic cocaine on offensive aggression. Low doses (15 and 30 mg/kg) of $MgCl_2$ and a Mg^{2+} deficiency maintain this inhibitory effect. As with chronic cocaine, 125 mg/kg $MgCl_2$ prevents a reduction in aggression following chronic haloperidol. These data support the notion that this high dose of $MgCl_2$ is maintaining catecholamine activity during drug treatments which reduce catecholamine activity (chronic cocaine and haloperidol).

Summary

Unlike tryptophan, Mg^{2+} alone has robust behavioral altering effects. These include elicitation of feeding, enhanced performance on a memory task, and facilitation of aggressive behavior. There is also an overlap between the behavioral effects of Mg^{2+} and stimulant drugs such as cocaine and amphetamine. A lack of specificity of the neurochemical mechanism of action of Mg^{2+} (i.e., it

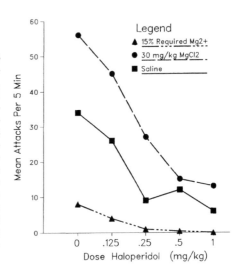

FIG. 6.4. Mean attacks per 5 min in male resident mice following various doses (0, .125, .25, .5 and 1 mg/kg) haloperidol and pretreatment with either saline (control), 30 mg/kg magnesium chloride (excess) or a 15% required magnesium diet (deficiency). Injections of haloperidol were made 60 min before testing and injections of saline or magnesium chloride were made 5 min before testing. The 15% required magnesium diet was fed for 3 weeks prior to testing. Drawn from Kantak, unpublished findings.

has an effect on diverse neurotransmitter systems) might preclude the therapeutic use of Mg^{2+} alone. Where a therapeutic benefit and specificity might be realized are with the combination of Mg^{2+} with other drugs which have a relatively specific mechanism of action. By enhancing or diminishing the potency of these drugs, Mg^{2+} cotreatment might offer some advantages over the use of these drugs alone. For example, stimulants are used to treat hyperactive children. If Mg^{2+} enhances the potency of stimulants, then less of the stimulant drug would be needed for clinical improvement. Another example is in the treatment of psychosis. By reducing the potency of haloperidol and preventing it's disruptive effects, Mg^{2+} might reduce the risk of developing tardive dyskinesia, yet permit clinical improvement for psychosis. The use of Mg^{2+} in this situation would be even more compelling if it can be demonstrated that Mg^{2+} prevents a D-2 receptor supersensitivity from developing in the nigrostriatal DA tract. This action has been demonstrated for Li^{2+} (Pert et al., 1979).

One final point concerns itself with the relative potency of Mg^{2+} with other divalent cations on receptor functions (Usdin et al., 1980). Although Mn^{2+} is slightly more potent than Mg^{2+} for these effects on receptors, Mn^{2+} is a trace mineral, i.e., it is needed in only very small amounts (microgram range). Toxicity can develop if too much is ingested (Cook, Fahn, & Brait, 1974). On the other hand, Mg^{2+} is not a trace mineral; it is needed in relatively high amounts (milligram range), and thus would be less likely to produce harmful effects than Mn^{2+}. Compared to Ca^{2+}, Mg^{2+} is more potent and compared to Li^{2+}, Mg^{2+} not only has the advantage of being more potent, but it also does not have as high a toxicity risk as Li^{2+}. The study of the behavioral interactions between Mg^{2+} and other mineral ions with drugs should prove to be interesting and fruitful.

ASCORBIC ACID

Ascorbic Acid Neurochemistry

The biological properties of ascorbic acid make it well suited for regulating numerous biochemical events (Bensch, Koerner, & Lohmann, 1981). In the brain, ascorbic acid may perform important functions related to the metabolism and release of several neurotransmitters. It is not synthesized in the brain, but is transported from the blood to the CSF (Spector, 1977; Vilter, 1967). Dopamine-beta-hydroxylase utilizes ascorbate as a cofactor which would have an impact on NE levels in noradrenergic neurons (Nakashima, Suzve, Kawada, & Samada, 1970). In addition, ascorbate inhibits the methylation of NE to normetanephrine, thus interfering with the catabolism of NE (Galzigna, Maina, & Rumney, 1971). There is an indirect role for ascorbate in the hydroxylation of tyrosine and tryptophan (Kaufman & Friedman, 1965), and it can stimulate the release of NE and ACH (Subramanian, 1977). In scorbutic guinea pigs, there is a large elevation in tyrosine ($+83\%$) and depressions in histidine (-33%) and GABA (-12%) (Enwonwu, 1971). The elevation in tyrosine may be due to an impairment in tyrosine hydroxylase in scorbutic animals.

Microiontophoretic application of ascorbic acid causes an acceleration in the firing rate of approximately one-third of the neurons tested in the anteromedial neostriatum (Gardiner et al., 1985). When ejected in conjunction with glutamic acid, this number is enhanced to two-thirds.

Receptor binding studies indicate that ascorbate decreases ligand binding to neurotransmitter receptors (Leslie, Dunlap, & Cox, 1980). The major effect is a reduction in the number of ligand binding sites (B_{max}). Ascorbate produces an 82% decrease in opiate binding site, an 18% decrease in DA binding sites, a 20% decrease in muscarinic binding sites, and a 50% decrease in alpha-NE binding sites. These reductions in the number of binding sites are most likely related to the ability of ascorbate to catalyze lipid peroxide formation which in turn produces the deleterious effects on membrane function (Schaefer, Komlos, & Seregi, 1975).

Ascorbic acid is a potent inhibitor of the binding of both DA agonists (^{3}H-dopamine and ^{3}H-ADTN) and DA antagonists (^{3}H-spiroperidol and ^{3}H-domperidone) to neostriatal membrane preparations (Heikkila, Cabbot, & Manzino, 1981). The relationship between ascorbate and DA agonist binding is a linear function where the higher the dose of ascorbic acid (up to 6 mM maximum concentration used) the greater the inhibition of binding. For DA antagonists, the relationship is an inverted—U function where at the lowest (0.006 mM) and highest (6 mM) concentrations used, inhibition of binding is found. There is little inhibitory effect at the two intermediated concentrations used (0.06 and 0.6 mM). The nature of the effect of ascorbic acid on the binding of DA agonists is quite different from its effect on the binding of DA antagonists. Additionally, ascorbate has an enhancing influence on presynaptic neurotransmitter mecha-

161

nisms, while the postsynaptic influence of ascorbate is inhibitory. Interestingly, this is the opposite relationship for magnesium.

Behavioral Effects of Ascorbic Acid Modulation

The preferential distribution of ascorbic acid in the brain and its effects on neurotransmitter mechanisms suggest that it may be involved in some central behavioral functions. By itself, ascorbic acid often fails to exert significant behavioral effects (e.g., Rebec, Centore, White, & Alloway, 1985). However, one noteworthy study using lower doses than are commonly used, found significant behavioral effects of ascorbic acid in rats which correlated with EEG activity (Wambebe & Sokomba, 1986). In a dose range of 50–400 mg/kg, ascorbic acid activated locomotion by 257% to 350%. The EEG of the frontal cortex and optic cortex were desynchronized while the EMG activity was slightly enhanced by the same dose range of ascorbate. These data suggest that ascorbate exerts stimulatory effects in rats. The discrepancy with other studies might be related to dose (low vs. high) and behavioral measurement (locomotion vs. stereotypy).

Clinical studies suggest a more robust role for ascorbate in altering behavior. It was reported by Horwitt in 1942 and by later investigators that schizophrenic patients receiving the usual dietary amounts of ascorbic acid had lower concentrations of ascorbic acid in the blood than people in good health. More recently, Pauling (1971) found that of the 106 schizophrenic patients studied, 81 (76%) were deficient in ascorbic acid, as shown by a 6 hr excretion of less than 17% of an orally administered dose. Only 27 of 89 control subjects (30%) showed this deficiency. However in another study, following a loading test of 500 mg ascorbate, no differences were found in blood levels between 32 schizophrenics and 24 demented control subjects (Pitt & Pollitt, 1971).

A significant controlled trial of ascorbic acid in chronic psychiatric patients was reported in 1963 by Milner. The study, which was double-blind, was made with 40 chronic male patients: 34 had schizophrenia, 4 had manic-depressive bipolar illness, and 2 had general paresis. Twenty of the patients, selected at random, received 1 gram of ascorbic acid per day for 3 weeks; the rest received a placebo. The patients were checked with the Minnesota Multiphasic Personality Inventory (MMPI) and the Wittenborn Psychiatric Rating Scale (WPRS) before and after the trial. It was concluded that statistically significant improvement in the depression, mania, and paranoid symptom-complexes, together with an improvement in overall personality functions, was obtained following saturation with ascorbic acid.

These studies indicate that ascorbic acid deficiency may be an important factor in the pathophysiology of schizophrenia and other dementias. Given the potent interactions between ascorbic acid and the dopamine system (see below), this hypothesis for a cause and treatment of schizophrenia deserves more serious attention.

Interactions with Ascorbic Acid and Drugs

Pretreatment with 500 mg/kg ascorbic acid, 30 min before the test drug, antagonizes the behavioral effects of LSD (50 ug/kg) and apomorphine (4 mg/kg), but not 5-Meo-DMT (100 ug/kg) on the limb flick response and abortive grooming response in cats (Trulson, Crisp, & Henderson, 1985). The fact that pretreatment with ascorbic acid does not change the behavioral response to 5-MEO-DMT is consistent with the finding that ascorbate does not interact with 5-HT binding sites, but does with DA sites. In this study, ascorbic acid alone produced no significant changes.

Haloperidol has been tested for its ability to block the behavioral response to amphetamine and to elicit catalepsy in rats treated with saline or 1000 mg/kg ascorbic acid (Rebec et al., 1985). By itself ascorbic acid fails to exert significant behavioral effects, but enhances the antiamphetamine (1 mg/kg) and cataleptogenic effect of haloperidol (0.1 or 0.5 mg/kg). The behavioral response to amphetamine included locomotion, rearing, sniffing, forelimb shuffling, and repetitive head movements. The largest effects were in the DA mediated stereotyped responses. Higher doses of ascorbic acid (1 to 2 g/kg) block the amphetamine response directly (Heikkila et al., 1981; Tolbert, Thomas, Middaugh, & Zemp, 1979). In contrast, Wambebe and Sokomba (1986) demonstrated that lower doses of ascorbic acid (100–200 mg/kg) significantly potentiate the behavioral excitation induced by 2.5 mg/kg d-amphetamine by approximately 75%. Catalepsy induced by 0.25 mg/kg haloperidol is attenuated by 50–200 mg/kg ascorbic acid.

Summary

The behavioral activating properties of low doses of ascorbic acid, either alone or in combination with stimulants, may be related to the large reduction in antagonist binding ability relative to agonist binding ability with low concentrations of ascorbic acid (Fig. 6.5). Under these conditions, effects of the antagonist haloperidol should be, and are, inhibited. With moderate or higher concentrations of ascorbic acid, agonist binding ability is reduced relative to antagonist binding ability. Thus, it would be expected that higher doses of ascorbic acid would decrease stimulant action and enhance neuroleptic action. Again, like the effects on neurotransmitter mechanisms, these effects of ascorbic acid are opposite those of magnesium.

CONCLUSIONS

Nutrients such as tryptophan, magnesium, and ascorbic acid have behavioral altering effects and alter the potency of certain specific drugs. What other nutrients exert such robust effects? It would not be too surprising to find that many

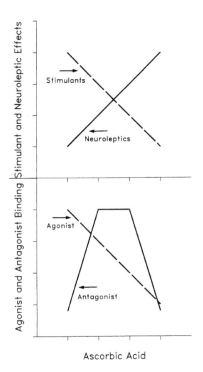

FIG. 6.5. Schematic drawing showing the effects of increasing concentrations of ascorbic acid on dopamine agonist and antagonist binding and its relationship to the behavioral actions of stimulants and neuroleptics following increasing doses of ascorbic acid. Derived from data described in Heikkila et al. (1984); Rebec et al. (1985) and Wambebe and Sokomba (1986).

nutrients are capable of such interactions. However, discovering which nutrients are the most potent and least toxic remains an arduous task. Since Dietary Behavioral Pharmacology is a new field, the first step would be to find out which nutrients are neurobiologically significant and behaviorally relevant. These types of studies would rely heavily upon the methods and procedures commonly used by Behavioral Pharmacologists and Neuropharmacologists.

Where will this new field lead us? Review of the previous studies indicates that the use of nutrients may represent a new therapeutic approach for a variety of brain related disorders. It is unlikely that a single nutrient alone would be effective in the treatment of a particular disorder. The most likely benefits would probably come from the combination of nutrients with drugs which have relatively specific mechanisms of action. By increasing the potency of drugs, this type of combined treatment might reduce the appearance of side effects, as well as reduce the development of tolerance and dependence on a drug because less drug would be needed. By decreasing the potency of drugs, certain toxic effects of drugs may be reduced or eliminated when given in conjunction with a nutrient.

Another possibility for therapeutic benefits is the use of a combination of nutrients as is used in some cases of autism where Mg^{2+} and vitamin B_6 are given. For example, would it be possible to titrate DA function with Mg^{2+} and ascorbic acid? This could be of use for Parkinson's Disease, Schizophrenia, Tardive Dyskinesia, Cocaine Abuse, and Attention Deficit Disorder, which are thought to be related to abnormal DA function. Data such as those reported here, indicate that the acute behavioral effects of diet should be taken seriously and should continue to be scientifically studied.

ACKNOWLEDGMENT

I want to thank Mary Ruth Fritz for her many volunteer hours doing literature searches in preparation for this manuscript.

REFERENCES

Aikawa, J. K. (1971). The biochemical and cellular functions of magnesium. In J. Durlach (Ed.), *1st International Symposium on Magnesium Deficit in Human Pathology* (pp. 39–56). France: Vittel.

Ashcroft, G. W., Crawford, T. B., Eccleston, D., Sharman, D. F., MacDougal, E. J., Stanton, J. B., & Binnis, J. K. (1966). 5-Hydroxyindole compounds in cerebrospinal fluid of patients with psychiatric or neurological diseases. *Lancet, 2,* 1049–1051.

Barthelemy, C., Garreau, B., Leddet, I., Ernouf, D., Muh, J. P., & LeLord, G. (1981). Behavioral and biological effects of oral magnesium, vitamin B_6 and combined magnesium-vitamin B_6 administration in autistic children. *Magnesium, 3,* 23–24.

Bensch, K. G., Koerner, O., & Lohmann, W. (1981). On a possible mechanism of action of ascorbic acid-formation of ionic bonds with biological molecules. *Biochemical and Biophysical Research Communications, 101,* 312–316.

Blasberg, R., & Lajtha, A. (1965). Substrate specificity of steady state amino acid transport in mouse brain slices. *Archives in Biochemistry and Biophysics, 112,* 361–377.

Boadle-Biber, M. C. (1978). Activation of tryptophan hydroxylase from central serotonergic neurons by calcium and depolarization. *Biochemical Pharmacology, 27,* 1069–1079.

Borbely, A. A., Neuhaus, H. U., & Tobler, I. (1981). Effect of parachlorophenylalanine and tryptophan on sleep, EEG and motor activity. *Behavioral Brain Research, 2,* 1–22.

Brown, G. L., Ebert, M. H., Goyer, P. F., Jimerson, D. C., Klein, W. J., Bunney, W. E., & Goodwin, F. K. (1982). Aggression, suicide and serotonin—relationships to CSF amine metabolites. *American Journal of Psychiatry, 139,* 741–746.

Brown, G. L., Goodwin, F. K., Bellenger, J. C., & Goyer, P. F. (1981). Cerebrospinal fluid amine metabolites and cyclic nucleotides in human aggression. *Psychopathology and Behavior, 17,* 63–65.

Carlsson, A., Davis, J. N., Kehr, W., Lindquist, M., & Attack, C. V. (1972). Simultaneous measurement of tyrosine and tryptophan hydroxylase activities in brain in vivo using an inhibitor of the aromatic amino acid decarboxylase. *Naunyn-Schmiedeberg's Archives of Pharmacology, 277,* 1–12.

Chouinard, G., Young, S. N., Annable, L., Sourkes, T. L. (1979). Tryptophan-nicotinamide, imipramine and their combination in depression—a controlled study. *Archives of Psychiatry Scandinavia, 59,* 395–414.

Chutkow, J. G., & Tyce, G. M. (1979). Brain norepinephrine, dopamine and 5-hydroxytryptamine in magnesium-deprivation encephalopathy in rats. *Journal of Neural Transmission, 44,* 297–302.

Colmenares, J. L., Wurtman, R. J., & Fernstrom, J. K. (1975). Effects of ingestion of a carbohydrate—fat meal on the levels and synthesis of 5-hydroxyindoles in various regions of the rat central nervous system. *Journal of Neurochemistry, 25,* 825–829.

Cook, D. G., Fahn, S., & Brait, K. A. (1974). Chronic manganese intoxication. *Archives of Neurology, 30,* 59–64.

Cooper, A. J., & Datta, S. R. (1980). A placebo controlled evaluation of L-tryptophan in depression in the elderly. *Canadian Journal of Psychiatry, 25,* 386–390.

Coppen, A., Shaw, D. M., & Farrell, J. P. (1963). Potentiation of the antidepressive effect of a monoamine oxidase inhibitor by tryptophan. *Lancet, 1,* 79–81.

Coppen, A., Shaw, D. M., Herzberg, B., & Maggs, R. (1967). Tryptophan in treatment of depression. *Lancet, 2,* 1178–1180.

Curzon, G., Joseph, M. H., & Knott, P. J. (1972). Effects of immobilization and food deprivation on rat brain tryptophan metabolism. *Journal of Neurochemistry, 19,* 1967–1974.

Dackis, C. A., & Gold, M. S. (1984). New concepts in cocaine addiction—the dopamine depletion hypothesis. *Neuroscience and Biobehavioral Reviews, 9,* 469–477.

DeVries, D. J., & Beart, P. M. (1985). Magnesium ions reveal nanomolar potency of dopamine at [3H] spiperone labelled D-2 receptors in rat corpus striatum. *European Journal of Pharmacology, 109,* 417–419.

Dews, P. (1986). Dietary pharmacology. *Nutritional Reviews, 44,* 246–251.

Enwonwu, C. O. (1971). Alterations in ninhydrin-positive substances and cytoplasmic protein synthesis in brains of ascorbic acid deficient guinea-pigs. *Journal of Neurochemistry, 21,* 69–78.

Essman, W. B. (1980). Cerebral hypomagnesemia and seizure susceptibility interdependence of 5-hydroxytryptamine metabolism. In M. Cantin & M. S. Seelig (Eds.), *Magnesium in health and disease* (pp. 785–790). New York: Spectrum.

Fernstrom, J. D., & Hirsch, M. J. (1975). Rapid depletion of brain serotonin in malnourished rats following 1-tryptophan injection. *Life Sciences, 17,* 455–464.

Fernstrom, J. D., & Jacoby, J. H. (1975). The interaction of diet and drugs in modifying brain serotonin metabolism. *General Pharmacology, 6,* 253–258.

Fernstrom, J. D., & Wurtman, R. J. (1971). Brain serotonin content: physiological dependence on plasma tryptophan levels. *Science, 173,* 149–152.

Gallager, D. W., & Aghajanian, G. K. (1976). Inhibition of firing of raphe neurons by tryptophan and 5-hydroxytryptophan—blockade by inhibiting serotonin synthesis with RO44602. *Neuropharmacology, 15,* 149–156.

Galzigna, L., Maina, L., & Rumney, L. (1971). Role of L-ascorbic-acid in reversal of monoamine oxidase inhibition by caffeine. *Journal of Pharmacy and Pharmacology, 23,* 303–305.

Gardiner, T. W., Armstrong, J. M., Caan, A. W., Wightman, R. M., & Rebec, G. V. (1985). Modulation of neostriatal activity by iontophoresis of ascorbic acid. *Brain Research, 344,* 181–185.

Gibbons, J. L., Barr, G. A., Bridger, W. H., & Leibowitz, S. F. (1979). Manipulations of dietary tryptophan: effects on mouse killing and brain serotonin in the rat. *Brain Research, 169,* 139–154.

Gibbons, J. L., Potegal, M., Blau, A. D., Ross, S., & Glusman, M. (1980). Quipazine and metergoline alter threshold for septal inhibition of muricide. *Society for Neuroscience Abstracts, 6,* 366.

Glossman, H., Hornung, R., & Presek, P. (1980). The use of ligand—binding for the characterization of alpha-adrenoceptors. *Journal of Cardiovascular Pharmacology, 2,* 303–324.

Grahame-Smith, D. G. (1971). Studies in vivo on the relationship between brain tryptophan, brain 5-HT synthesis and hyperactivity in rats treated with a monoamine oxidase inhibitor and L-tryptophan. *Journal of Neurochemistry, 18,* 1053–1066.

Griffiths, W. J., Lester, B. K., & Coulter, J. D. (1972). Tryptophan and sleep in young adults. *Psychophysiology, 9,* 345–356.

Hamblin, M. W., & Creese, I. (1982). 3H-Dopamine binding to rat striatal D-2 and D-3 sites:

enhancement by magnesium and inhibition by guanine nucleotides and sodium. *Life Sciences, 30,* 1587–1595.

Hartman, E., & Greenwald, D. (1984). L-tryptophan and sleep. In H. G. Schlossberger, W. Kochen, B. Linzen, & H. Steinhart (Eds.), *Progress in Tryptophan and Serotonin Research* (pp. 297–304). Berlin: Walter de Gruyter & Company.

Heikkila, R. E., Cabbat, F. S., & Manzino, L. (1981). Differential inhibitory effects of ascorbic acid on the binding of dopamine agonists and antagonists to neostriatal membrane preparations: correlations with behavioral effects. *Research Communications in Chemical Pathology and Pharmacology, 34,* 409–421.

Herrington, R. N., Bruce, A., Johnston, E. C., & Lader, M. H. (1976). Comparative trial of L-tryptophan and amitriptyline in depressive illness. *Psychological Medicine, 6,* 673–678.

Hole, K., & Marsden, C. A. (1975). Unchanged sensitivity to electric shock in L-tryptophan treated rats. *Pharmacology, Biochemistry and Behavior, 3,* 307–309.

Horwitt, M. K. (1942). Ascorbic acid requirement of individuals in a large institution. *Proceedings of the Society for Experimental Biology and Medicine, 49,* 248–250.

Izenwasser, S. I., Garcia-Valdez, K., & Kantak, K. M. (1986). Stimulant-like effects of magnesium on aggression in mice. *Pharmacology Biochemistry and Behavior, 25,* 1195–1199.

Kakiuchi, S., Yamazaki, R., & Teshima, Y. (1972). Regulation of brain phosphodiesterase activity: Ca^{2+} plus Mg^{2+}—dependent phosphodiesterase and its activating factor from rat brain. In P. Greengard, G. A. Robison, & R. Paoletti, (Eds.), *Advances in cyclic nucleotide research, Vol. 1,* (pp. 455–477). New York: Raven Press.

Kanoff, P. D., Hegstrand, L. R., & Greengard, P. (1977). Biochemical characterization of histamine-sensitive adenylate cyclase in mammalian brain. *Archives in Biochemistry and Biophysics, 182,* 321–334.

Kantak, K. M. (1986). Changes in cocaine potency with magnesium excess and deficiency. *Society for Neuroscience Abstracts, 12,* 920.

Kantak, K. M. (1988). Magnesium deficiency alters aggressive behavior and catecholamine function. *Behavioral Neuroscience, 102,* 304–311.

Kantak, K. M., & Adlerstein, L. K. (1985). Alteration in catecholamine function with magnesium. *Society for Neuroscience Abstracts, 11,* 670.

Kantak, K. M., Hegstrand, L. R., & Eichelman, B. (1980b). Dietary tryptophan modulation and aggressive behavior in mice. *Pharmacology, Biochemistry and Behavior, 12,* 675–679.

Kantak, K. M., Hegstrand, L. R., & Eichelman, B. (1981). Dietary tryptophan reversal of septal lesion and 5,7-DHT lesion elicited shock-induced fighting. *Pharmacology Biochemistry and Behavior, 15,* 343–350.

Kantak, K. M., Hegstrand, L. R., Whitman, J., & Eichelman, B. (1980a). Effects of dietary supplements and a tryptophan-free diet on aggressive behavior. *Pharmacology, Biochemistry and Behavior, 12,* 173–179.

Kantak, K. M., Wayner, M. J., & Stein, J. M. (1978). Effects of various periods of food deprivation on serotonin synthesis in the lateral hypothalamus. *Pharmacology Biochemistry and Behavior, 9,* 535–541.

Kaufman, S. (1974). Properties of pterin-dependent aromatic amino acid hydroxylase. In G. E. W. Wolstenholme & D. W. Fitzsimons (Eds.), *Aromatic amino acids in the brain* (pp. 85–115). Amsterdam: Associated Scientific.

Kaufman, S., & Friedman, S. (1965). Dopamine—Beta—Hydroxylase. *Pharmacology Reviews, 17,* 71–107.

Kruesi, M. J. P. (1986). Diet and human behavior: How much do they affect each other? *Annual Review of Nutrition, 6,* 113–130.

Landfield, P. W., & Morgan, G. A. (1984). Chronically elevating plasma Mg^{2+} improves hippocampal frequency potentiation and reversal learning in aged and young rats. *Brain Research, 322,* 167–171.

Leccese, H. P., & Lyness, W. H. (1984). The effects of putative 5-hydroxytryptamine receptor active agents on d-amphetamine self-administration in controls and rats with 5,7-dihydroxytryptamine medial forebrain bundle lesions. *Brain Research, 303,* 153–162.

Lefkowitz, R. J., Mullikin, D., & Caron, M. G. (1976). Regulation of B-adrenergic receptors by guanyl-5'-yl imidodiphosphate and other purine nucleotides. *Journal of Biological Chemistry, 15,* 4686–4692.

LeLord, G., Callaway, E., & Muh, J. P. (1982). Clinical and biological effects of high doses of vitamin B_6 and magnesium on autistic children. *Acta Vitaminologia et Enzymologica, 4,* 27–44.

Leslie, F. M., Dunlap, C. E., & Cox, B. M. (1980). Ascorbate decreases ligand binding to neurotransmitter receptors. *Journal of Neurochemistry, 34,* 219–221.

Lieberman, H. R. (1986). Behavioral changes caused by nutrients. *Bibl. Nutr. Dieta., 38,* 219–224.

Lyness, W. A. (1983). Effect of l-tryptophan pretreatment on d-amphetamine self-administration. *Substance and Alcohol Actions/Misuse, 4,* 305–312.

Martineau, J., Barthelemy, C., Garreau, B., & LeLord, G. (1985). Vitamin B_6, magnesium and combined B_6—Mg: therapeutic effects in childhood autism. *Biological Psychiatry, 20,* 465–468.

McMenamy, R., & Oncley, J. (1958). The specific bindings of L-tryptophan to serum albumin. *Journal of Biological Chemistry, 233,* 1436–1442.

Messing, R. B., Fisher, L. A., Phebus, L., & Lytle, L. D. (1976). Interaction of diet and drugs in the regulation of brain 5-hydroxyindoles and response to painful electric shock. *Life Sciences, 18,* 707–714.

Milner, G. (1963). Ascorbic acid in chronic psychiatric patients: a controlled trial. *Brittish Journal of Psychiatry, 109,* 294–299.

Moller, S. E., Kirk, L., & Fremming, K. H. (1976). Plasma amine acids as an index for subgroups in manic-depressive psychosis-correlation to effect of tryptophan. *Psychopharmacology, 49,* 205–213.

Morand, C., Young, S. N., & Ervin, F. R. (1983). Clinical response of aggressive schizophrenics to oral tryptophan. *Biological Psychiatry, 18,* 575–578.

Murphy, D. L., Baker, M., Goodwin, F. K., Miller, H., Kotin, J., & Bunney, W. E. (1974). L-tryptophan in affective disorders-indoleamine changes and differential clinical effects. *Psychopharmacology, 34,* 11–20.

Nakashima, Y., Suzve, R., Kawada, S., & Samada, H. (1970). Effects of ascorbic acid in hydroxylase activity. 1. Stimulation of tyrosine hydroxylase and tryptophan—5 hydroxylase activities by ascorbic acid. *Journal of Vitaminology, 16,* 276–280.

Nelson, D. L., Herbet, A., Enjalbert, A., Bockaert, J., & Hamon, M. (1980). Serotonin—sensitive adenylate cyclase and [^{3}H] serotonin binding sites in the CNS of the rat—I. *Biochemical Pharmacology, 29,* 2445–2453.

Pare, C. M. (1963). Potentiation of monoamine-oxidase inhibitors by tryptophan. *Lancet, 2,* 527–528.

Pasternak, G. W., Snowman, A. M., & Snyder, S. H. (1975). Selective enhancement of (^{3}H) opiate agonist binding by divalent cations. *Molecular Pharmacology, 11,* 735–744.

Pauling, L. (1971). On the orthomolecular environment of the mind: Orthomolecular theory. *American Journal of Psychiatry, 133,* 1251–1257.

Pert. A., Rosenblatt, J. E., Sivit, C., Pert, C. B., & Bunney, W. E. (1979). Long-term treatment with lithium prevents the development of dopamine receptor supersensitivity. *Science, 201,* 171–173.

Pitt, B., & Pollitt, N. (1971). Ascorbic acid and chronic schizophrenia. *Brittish Journal of Psychiatry, 118,* 227–228.

Raese, J. D., Edelman, A. M., Makk, G., Bruckwich, E. A., Lovenberg, W., & Barchas, J. D. (1979). Brain striatal tyrosine hydroxylase: activation of the enzyme by AMP-independent phosphorylation. *Communications in Psychopharmacology, 3,* 295–301.

Rebec, G. V., Centore, J. M., White, L. K., & Alloway, K. D. (1985). Ascorbic acid and the behavioral response to haloperidol: Implications for the action of antipsychotic drugs. *Science, 227,* 438–440.

Rouot, B. M., U'Prichard, D. C., & Snyder, S. H. (1980). Multiple alpha-2 noradrenergic receptor sites in rat brain: selective regulation of high affinity ^{3}H-clonidine binding by guanine nucleotides and divalent cations. *Journal of Neurochemistry, 34,* 374–384.

Schaefer, A., Komlos, M., & Seregi, A. (1975). Lipid peroxidation as the cause of the ascorbic acid induced decrease of adenosine triphosphate activities of rat brain microsomes and its inhibition by biogenic amines and psychotropic drugs. *Biochemical Pharmacology, 24,* 1781–1786.

Seoane, J. R., Cote, M., & Liretto, A. (1981). Effects of intraventricular injections of Ca^{2+} and (or) Mg^{2+} on eating behavior, water intake and cardiac rhythm in sheep. *Journal of Animal Science, 53,* 317–322.

Simmons, K. (1985). Scientists ponder diets behavioral effects. *Journal of the American Medical Association, 254,* 3407–3408.

Smith, F. L., Yu, D. S. L., Smith, D. G., Leceese, A. P., & Lyness, W. H. (1986). Dietary tryptophan supplements attenuate amphetamine self-administration in the rat. *Pharmacology, Biochemistry, and Behavior, 25,* 849–855.

Spector, R. (1977). Vitamin homeostasis in the central nervous system. *New England Journal of Medicine, 296,* 1393–1398.

Spinweber, C. L., Ursin, R., Hilbert, R. P., & Hilderbrand, R. L. (1983). L-tryptophan: effects on daytime sleep latency EEG. *Electroencephalography and Clinical Neurophysiology, 55,* 652–661.

Subramanian, N. (1977). Brain ascorbic acid and its importance in metabolism of biogenic amines. *Life Sciences, 20,* 1479–1484.

Tagliamonte, A., Tagliamonte, P., Perez-Cruet, J., & Gessa, G. (1972). Control of male sexual behavior by monoaminergic and cholinergic mechanisms. *Psychopharmacology, 26,* 131–141.

Tolbert, L. C., Thomas, T. N., Middaugh, L. D., & Zemp, J. W. (1979). Effect of ascorbic acid on neurochemical, behavioral and physiological systems mediated by catecholamines. *Life Sciences, 25,* 2189–2195.

Traskman, K., Asberg, M., Bertilsson, L., & Sjostrand, L. (1981). Monoamine metabolites in CSF and suicide behavior. *Archives of General Psychiatry, 38,* 631–636.

Trulson, M. E., Crisp, T., & Henderson, L. J. (1985). Ascorbic acid antagonizes the behavioral effects of LSD in cats. *Journal of Pharmacy and Pharmacology, 37,* 930–931.

Udenfriend, S., Titus, E., Weissbach, H., & Peterson, R. E. (1956). Biogenesis and metabolism of 5-hydroxyindole compounds. *Journal of Biological Chemistry, 219,* 335–344.

Udenfriend, S., & Weissbach, H. (1958). Turnover of 5-hydroxytryptamine (serotonin) in tissue. *Proceedings of the Society for Experimental Biology, 97,* 748–751.

Usdin, T. B., Creese, I., & Snyder, S. H. (1980). Regulation by cations of [^{3}H] spiroperidol binding associated with dopamine receptors of rat brain. *Journal of Neurochemistry, 34,* 669–676.

Vilter, R. W. (1967). Pharmacology. In W. H. Sebrell & R. S. Harris (Eds.), *The vitamins* (pp. 487–490). New York: Academic Press.

Walters, J. K., Davis, M., & Sheard, M. H. (1979). Tryptophan-free diet effects on the acoustic startle reflex in rats. *Psychopharmacology 62,* 103–109.

Wambebe, C., & Sokomba, E. (1986). Some behavioral and EEG effects of ascorbic acid in rats. *Psychopharmacology, 89,* 167–170.

Watanabe, M., George, S. R., & Seeman, P. (1985). Regulation of anterior pituitary D-2 receptors by magnesium and sodium ions. *Journal of Neurochemistry, 45,* 1842–1849.

Weinberger, S. B., Knapp, S., & Mandell, A. J. (1978). Failure of tryptophan load-induced increases in brain serotonin to alter food intake in the rat. *Life Sciences, 22,* 1595–1602.

Williams L. T., Mullikin, D., & Lefkowitz, R. J. (1978). Magnesium dependence of agonist binding to adenylate cyclase-coupled hormone receptors. *Journal of Biological Chemistry, 253,* 29984–2989.

Young, S. N. (1986). The effect on aggression and mood of altering tryptophan levels. *Nutritional Reviews, 44,* 112–122.

7 Roles and Characteristics of Theory in Behavioral Pharmacology

Marc N. Branch
David W. Schaal
University of Florida, Gainesville

Behavioral pharmacology has existed as an identifiable scientific discipline for more than 30 years (Branch, 1984; Pickens, 1977). Over that time a large array of data has been collected as witnessed by the series in which this chapter appears and other compendia (e.g., Blackman & Sanger, 1978; Efron, 1968; Seiden & Balster, 1985; Thompson, Pickens, & Meisch, 1970). Yet to be developed, however, is a coherent theoretical framework that provides organization for that array. This chapter, lamentably, does not provide such a theory, but we hope it will help provide a base for the development of a theory (or theories) for behavioral pharmacology. To that end, the major purpose of the chapter is to provide a framework that illustrates what a theory for behavioral pharmacology should entail.

The chapter is divided into four major sections. The first deals with the question, "What should the theory be about?" Perhaps the question could be restated as, "What is behavioral pharmacology?" The second section describes the nature and characteristics of theories in general. Here, issues of prediction, explanation and the role of reductionism are discussed. The third part describes, briefly, the nature of behavioral theory that has emerged from the subdiscipline within psychology known as the experimental analysis of behavior. It is argued that some of this theory is especially well suited to serve both as a model and as a basis for theory in behavioral pharmacology. The last section outlines the major characteristics that theory for behavioral pharmacology might take. In this section, not only is behavioristic theory utilized as a model for theory development, but, in addition, a role to be played by pharmacological theory is delineated.

171

THE DOMAIN OF BEHAVIORAL PHARMACOLOGY

Before one can begin to develop a theory, some judgment must be exercised as to what the theory is to describe and explain. That is, the range of natural phenomena to be dealt with must be circumscribed. As it turns out, this is not a simple problem in the case of behavioral pharmacology because there has not been, and there is not now, uniform agreement as to what the discipline entails. The range of possibilities is illustrated by differences among definitions that one finds in textbooks purporting to focus on behavioral pharmacology. In the original textbook for the field (Thompson & Schuster, 1968), it was proposed that behavioral pharmacology represented the wedding of two scientific disciplines, pharmacology and experimental psychology (especially the experimental analysis of behavior), and that its focus should be on explanation of the *behavioral* (italics mine) actions of drugs. That is, explanations should not be based on mental or neural events. In this way, *behavioral* pharmacology could be viewed as distinct from its cousins psychopharmacology and neuropharmacology.

Later textbooks, however, included definitions that do not separate behavioral pharmacology from the domains of psycho- or neuro-pharmacology. For example, Glick and Goldfarb (1976) stated that behavioral pharmacology, the study of the interactions of drugs with behavior, has three aims: (1) to use behavior as an indicator to examine drug effects, with the focus on differentiating drug classes; (2) to use behavior as an indicator to make inferences about the neurochemical processes that "underlie" behavior; (3) to develop screening procedures to identify clinically useful compounds. Another example is provided by Iversen and Iversen (1981) who essentially state simply that behavioral pharmacology is the study of drugs that influence behavior. In other words, behavioral pharmacology could include the study of effects of amphetamine (a drug that can influence behavior) on isolated brain slices.

The divergence of opinion concerning a definition for behavioral pharmacology continues to the present and is illustrated by the definitions presented in the two most recent textbooks in the field. Carlton (1983) defines the field in much the same way that Thompson and Schuster (1968) did. He proposes that the discipline be focused on analyzing the behavioral mechanisms of drug action. By contrast, McKim (1986) suggests that behavioral pharmacology refers to the study of behaviorally active drugs across a variety of levels of investigation.

It is clear from the foregoing that, at least among authors of textbooks, there is no firm guidance as to what the domain of behavioral pharmacology is. An examination of the origins of the field and its subsequent development, however, may provide a better guide.

Although it was the clinical success of chlorpromazine in the treatment of psychotic disorders during the early 1950s that gave initial impetus to the study of behaviorally active drugs (a broad enterprise that is referred to here as psychopharmacology), it was the pioneering research of P. B. Dews that gave rise to the expression "behavioral pharmacology." It is with his work, then, that the discipline that is the focus of this chapter began. Dews (e.g., 1955, 1956) showed that the behavioral action of a drug can depend on the circumstances responsible for the behavior. For example, he found (Dews, 1955) that a particular dose of pentobarbital could increase the probability of a particular activity (i.e., act as a "stimulant") or decrease the probability of that same activity (i.e., act as a "depressant") depending on subtle features of the environmental conditions responsible for the maintenance of the behavior. Subsequent to this exciting, and still puzzling, discovery, many reports illustrating that environmental factors can be crucial determinants of drug action appeared (for several illustrations see Thompson et al., 1970). And it was this literature and the research that generated it that constituted the field of behavioral pharmacology.

Attempts to provide theoretical integration of these findings included the concept of rate-dependency (Dews, 1958, 1964; Kelleher & Morse, 1968) and interpretations based on other behavioral processes (e.g., Dews & Morse, 1961). As these attempts subsequently were found to be of limited applicability (e.g., Branch & Gollub, 1974; Gonzalez & Byrd, 1977; McAuley & Leslie, 1986), however, greater reliance on reductionistic pharmacological interpretations developed. This change was spurred by two major developments. First, during the 1970s there was a dramatic increase in research on drugs as discriminative stimuli, with special emphasis on "generalization" across different drugs (Stolerman & Shine, 1985). That is, stimulus control would be established using one drug as a discriminative stimulus and then other drugs would be substituted to see if they had similar discriminative properties. Second, there was an explosive growth in knowledge about receptors with which various classes of drugs interacted (Snyder, 1984). For example, it was discovered that specific receptors exist to which opioids bind and through which they exert their effects (e.g., Martin et al., 1976). This second development helped to provide an interpretive framework for research on drug discrimination. Specifically, it was discovered that one can predict with some accuracy that drugs that exert similar discriminative control bind to the same receptor. The success of these types of interpretations served not only to show that behavioral techniques may be used to make pharmacological inferences, but also led to a great deal of emphasis on reductionistic, pharmacological interpretations of research on drug-behavior interactions in general. The shift in interpretive base predictably was accompanied by a shift in research emphases. Currently, research conducted under the rubric of behavioral pharmacology frequently is focused on pharmacological questions rather than behavioral ones (see Seiden & Balster, 1985). That is, what counts as behavioral pharmacology is no longer limited to research on environmental determination of drug action. Consequently, a comprehensive theory for the discipline most surely will have to include concepts from pharmacology, including the reductionistic concept of the receptor. Happily, receptor theory is comparatively well developed, so those aspects of behavioral pharmacology that are reductionistically oriented already have an established set of theoretical principles upon which to be based. But what of the case for the part of behavioral pharmacology that is not receptor oriented, but instead deals with the analysis of environmental determination of drug effects? We ought not to forget that there is a wealth of literature illustrating such effects, and that these provocative effects were the ones that gave birth to the discipline. It is this branch of behavioral pharmacology that is more in need of theory construction. It is clear that a complete theory for behavioral pharmacology must include explanations of these kinds of effects. This can be illustrated syllogistically:

> Premise 1: Different behavioral activities can be (and often are) affected differently by a drug.
> Premise 2: Different environments (this includes, of course, histories) can produce different behavioral activities and patterns of activities.
> Therefore: Different environments can produce different drug effects.

Theory is needed, therefore, to characterize and explain environmental/behavioral determination of drug action. The question that remains concerns what form this theory will take. Should its development be guided by the search for reductionistic mechanisms akin to receptors, or should some other strategy be employed? Before attempting to answer this question, it may be profitable to outline some of the basic characteristics of theories in general.

THEORIES: THEIR ROLES AND CHARACTERISTICS

Roles of Theories

Theories generally are recognized to serve two major roles: (a) a heuristic role, and (b) to serve as a basis for prediction and explanation. With regard to the latter Campbell (1920) has noted that *theory* in the language of science has come to designate "connected sets of propositions" which serve as the formal basis for the prediction and explanation of phenomena. Effective science, it has been argued, cannot exist in the absence of theory. Science is not simply the accumulation of facts even though such accumulation is essential. As stated by Poincaré (1909): "Experiment is the sole source of truth . . . it *alone* can give us certainty," but ". . . to observe is not enough. We must use our observations, and to do that we must generalize" (p. 167). "Science is built up with facts as a house is with stones. But a collection of facts is no more a science than a heap of stones is a house" (p. 167). That is, we need an organizational scheme into which to place our facts, and a question that arises concerns what should such a scheme be like. There is general agreement among philosophers of science that a theory should be as simple as possible. Poincaré (1909) argued that one should organize until "we have found simplicity" (p. 176). A major role of theory, then, is to organize experience in the simplest way possible that still allows us to speak accurately about the world, or as stated more eloquently by Mach (1960) who discussed the "economy of science," "Science itself, therefore, may be regarded as a minimal problem, consisting of the completest possible presentment of facts with the *least possible expenditure of thought*" (p. 586).

A theory, then, should be as simple as possible a source of prediction and explanation. The meaning of prediction is clear to most everyone, but explanation is another matter. Among philosophers of science, however, there is some agreement as to what constitutes explanation. Basically, a phenomenon has been "explained" when it can be shown that it represents an instance of some familiar, more general principle (Turner, 1965). Or, as Schlick (1949) has noted, explanation is the "discovery of the like in the unlike." A scientific law, therefore, can serve as an explanation. For example, an apple dropping from a tree and a rifle bullet fired from the top of a skyscraper (two seemingly unlike events) can be described by the "law" of gravitation. That is, the time it takes for each to hit the ground can be deduced from the same principle. These two events thus are seen to be alike as instances of a familiar principle (gravitational attraction) and are thus "explained." This kind of explanation (lawful explanation), however, can be viewed as inferior to theoretical explanation. A theory allows the derivation of laws and thus represents a more fundamental explanation. Taking a Machian view, knowing the basic tenets of the theory means you do not have to remember explicitly each of the laws that can be derived from them, and, therefore, knowing the theory is more economical, thoughtwise, than is knowing all the laws. Consequently, theoretical explanation is predicated on a simpler base. Note that explanation is *not* based on an account at some other level of analysis, i.e., reductionism is not required for explanation, even for theoretical explanation.

A second major role played by theory is a heuristic one. In extremely well-formulated theories theorems may be derived that serve as hypotheses to be tested experimentally. That is, the theory dictates which experiments are important to carry out. More generally, a theory prescribes a conceptual framework to view the work and, as such, determines the field of research (Turner, 1965). That this is true is illustrated by the brief historical outline presented earlier. Much of the current research in behavioral pharmacology is guided by receptor theory, and the lack of even a poorly developed theory concerning environmental determination of drug action has led to a curtailment of research in this important domain, partly because it is not clear what the important undone experiments are.

Characteristics of Theories

Although there is general agreement about what the major characteristics of theories are, there is some controversy over which characteristics are the most important for effective theories. One of the more controversial issues is the importance of "underlying reality."

One perspective is that "underlying reality" is the true essence of theory. For example, Turner (1965) argues that once something has been observed it is no longer theoretical, a view that is in accord with the dictionary meaning of the word. It is from the unobserved "underlying reality," or the presumptive hypotheses of the theory, that one derives the theorems to be examined experimentally. From this point of view, the major concern is not with the "truth" or "reality" of the presumptive hypotheses but with the truth of the derived theorems.

An alternative perspective has been described by the physicist Duhem (1954). He asserts that theories have two aspects, a representative, or descriptive, part and an explanatory part. The descriptive part of a theory consists of the simplest (à la Mach) possible description of the known relationships, whereas the explanatory part represents an attempt to take hold of "underlying reality." Duhem believed that the descriptive, or representative, part of a theory is more important. "Everything good in the theory, by virtue of which it appears as a natural classification and confers on it the power to *anticipate experience* is found in the representative part; all of what was discovered by the physicist while he forgot about the search for explanation" (p. 32, italics added). He did acknowledge, however, a modest heuristic role for the explanatory part albeit somewhat grudgingly when he noted that "Chimerical hopes may have incited admirable discoveries without these discoveries embodying the chimeras which gave birth of them. Bold explorations [in] geography are due to adventurers who were looking for the golden land; that is not sufficient reason for inscribing 'El Dorado' on our maps of the globe" (pp. 31–32).

The views espoused by Turner and Duhem really are not that different; both acknowledge a role for guesses about "underlying reality" and both also acknowledge the importance of the descriptive parts of theories (witness Turner's view on the importance of the "truth" of derived theorems). Their differences center around which aspect is more important. Turner is concerned that concentrating only on observables will take the "theoretical" out of theory. That worry is unfounded. Even the descriptive part of a theory contains much that is theoretical. That is, the descriptive part of a theory includes (either directly or via derivation) the laws that describe relationships between independent and dependent variables. For those relationships where these variables are continuous it is not possible (nor wise) to examine *every* value of the independent variable, so the effects of untested values remain truly theoretical. Thus, it is the descriptive part of a theory that is falsifiable. (Another important aspect of any theory is that it be falsifiable.) For example, evolutionary theory (its descriptive part) proposes that certain life forms preceded others through the history of the earth. Consequently, if one were to find the remains of a mammal that could be dated convincingly as 800 million years old, the theory would be seen to be false.

It may be a mistake to refer to the "underlying reality" or the presumptive hypotheses of a theory as the "explanatory" part. As noted earlier, explanation does not rest necessarily on some sort of underlying mechanisms; instead it rests on identifying phenomena as instances that fall into a familiar context(s). Recognition of this fact coupled with the realization that the descriptive aspect of a theory remains "theoretical" leads to the conclusion that presumptions or speculations about "underlying realities" are not a necessary part of theory.

Closely related to issues of underlying reality are those concerning the place of "reductionism" in theory and explanation. Is it the case that more encompassing theories are necessarily "reductionistic" when compared to more restricted theories? Before dealing with this thorny issue, and one that seems especially relevant to behavioral pharmacology (as well as to psychology in general), it may be helpful to follow the lead of Nagel (1949) with respect to distinguishing between two types of theoretical reduction. Nagel's two types of reduction are labeled homogeneous and nonhomogeneous. Homogeneous theoretical reduction presents no serious problem, for it represents cases in which the new, or reducing, theory has no new terms or entities when compared to the old, or reduced, theory. An example of a homogeneous reduction is the "reduction" of Galileo's laws of falling bodies to Newton's law of motion. Galileo's theory was reduced to Newton's in the sense that Newton's laws encompassed Galileo's and, as well, applied to a broader range of phenomena. A similar step was taken when Newton's laws were subsumed by relativity theory. In each case, the same phenomena were explained with the same basic set of terms. All deal with mass, distance and time as basic quantities. Homogeneous reductions illustrate the major advantage of reduction; a broader array of phenomena are encompassed without a corresponding increase in the number of explanatory principles. Thus, theoretical reduction exemplifies Mach's "economy of science." A *successful* reduction, then, is one that provides a *broader* account.

Nonhomogeneous reduction presents a more complicated problem because, here, new terms are introduced in the reducing science, and how these terms are to be "translated" into a form that allows the reduced science to be subsumed must be worked out. Nagel points to the reduction of classical thermodynamics to the kinetic theory of gases as an example of a successful nonhomogeneous reduction. It is important to note that thermodynamics was a very well documented and established descriptive theory *before* it was reduced. Kinetic theory was also well developed. Such development appears essential for a successful nonhomogeneous reduction, both so that correspondences may be observed and so that fundamental differences in terms may be identified. A major difference between thermodynamics and the kinetic theory is that the concept of "temperature" does not exist in the latter, whereas it plays a major role in the former. Thermodynamics is successfully reduced only when the mean kinetic energy of molecules is equated with temperature. This equation, Nagel argues, has the status of a hypothesis. It cannot be shown to be formally true. Thus, the successful nonhomogeneous reduction of thermodynamics to the kinetic theory of gases remains at its root, tentative (despite the enormous mass of data indicating that the reduction is "true.") This is in contrast to homogeneous reduction, where the laws of the reduced theory can be formally derived, without additional hypotheses, from the reducing theory. Despite the logical "flaw" in non-homogeneous reduction it remains true that success is defined in terms of being able to account for a broader range of phenomena.

Nagel's analysis of reduction has implications for theory development in behavioral pharmacology. As noted earlier, there currently is considerable emphasis given to neuropharmacological interpretation of experimental results in behavioral pharmacology. These interpretations may be assumed to be attempts at nonhomogeneous reductionistic theorizing, i.e., as attempts to explain phenomena that include behavioral components *via* neurochemical principles. Nagel's view suggests that this should be done with great caution (and perhaps ·with trepidation) because the behavioral phenomena have yet to be well characterized at their own level. That is, until behavioral theory is reasonably well-developed, it will not be possible to assess the utility of trying to reduce that theory to one based in neurophysiology.

There is another view of reductionism that is important for theory construction in behavioral pharmacology. This view may be termed *constitutive reductionism* (cf. Thompson, 1984). Behaving organisms are constructed of, or consist of, physiology. Obviously, therefore, when an organism behaves or is exposed to circumstances that alter how it behaves subsequently, its physiology must change. One way of stating this is to say that an organism's physiology *participates* in behavior. When thought of in this way, an organism's physiology is less likely to be thought of as the cause of behavior. Instead, the physiological changes are viewed as part of the changes that occur. In this sense, a description of physiological changes does not serve as an explanation of behavior, but instead provides a more complete account of the changes wrought by the "real" causes (e.g., drug administration, a particular set of experiences, etc.) That is, the physiological changes are effects, not causes. Of course, in a logical analysis the preceding argument falls short because, at least in some cases, physiological changes can be shown to be necessary and sufficient precursors to other physiological actions and behavioral responses. For pragmatic reasons, however, it is useful to have a theory that incorporates manipulable environmental events as independent variables. These reasons are discussed more fully in the section on behavioristic theory.

A final characteristic of theories that deserves brief mention is a theory's syntax or calculus. In physics that calculus is the language of mathematics, a language that allow no ambiguity. By contrast, any science concerned with behavior, as behavioral pharmacology is, currently is restricted to everyday speech. This presents a potentially serious problem because everyday language, e.g., English, often is not very precise, largely due to the sometimes varied and sometimes shared histories of those who speak the language. It is reasonable to assume that the effectiveness and usefulness of a calculus depends on the precision with which it is used. Hineline (1980, 1984) has emphasized this point as a reason for avoiding cognitive terms since many of them tend to be burdened with extra meaning. For example, a term like "retrieval," which in ordinary use means that someone went somewhere and removed something from a location, is not supposed to imply that (i.e., removal) when referring to behavioral processes involved in remembering. A counterargument is that as long as things are well operationalized no one will be misled. As Hineline notes, this argument seems to be based on the notion that past history can be rendered irrelevant. He offers an example of the following sort: You say to someone at a public gathering, "I operationally define 'jerk' as a sensitive, socially polished, intelligent, admirable person. You are a jerk!" It seems reasonable to assume that the effects on the listener, who has just been called a jerk, will depend not only on the operational definition but also on his or her previous history with respect to the word. That is, despite the operational definition, the jerk might be offended.

Problems of the sort just described can be avoided, and therefore unintended confusion can be avoided, by the development and use of a precise technical language. Just as physicists have invented terms like "quark," so, too, can those interested in behavior generate technical terms that have no counterpart in everyday speech. Consequently, one ought not be embarrassed by the use of a technical vocabulary but rather should see it as essential to effective progress. Paying attention to how one talks about behavior, therefore, is not merely a pedantic exercise. It may be crucial to the development of an effective theory for behavioral pharmacology. An emphasis on precision and accuracy is a hallmark of behavioristic theory within psychology, and it is to such theory that we now turn.

BEHAVIORISTIC THEORY

Behavioral pharmacology has relied heavily on the methods developed in the experimental analysis of behavior. These methods generally are agreed to be the most powerful yet developed for the study of behavioral processes. These techniques, interestingly, have their origin in behavioristic theory. If the theory has led to the development of the best methods available (as we argue it has), then perhaps it also may provide the best available starting point in an attempt to develop a theory about the behavioral effects of drugs.

Behavioristic theory has many important characteristics, only a few of which are touched upon here. (For an impressively complete treatment, see Zuriff, 1985.) Those selected are those that are most relevant to behavioral pharmacology.

Behavioristic theory is predicated initially on the belief that the study of behavior falls in the realm of the natural sciences, and therefore that the goals of such a theory include prediction and control of natural phenomena. Also attendent to such a belief is the notion of the unity of science; that physics, chemistry, biology and the science of behavior (and others), in addition to sharing the same goals (prediction and control), also are not mutually exclusive, but deal with different aspects of nature. The idea here is that chemistry involves physics, biology involves chemistry, etc., yet each discipline can stand on its own due to the type of phenomena under investigation. Behavioristic theory is predicated on the belief that behavior, in its own right, is a proper subject matter for science. Behavior, then, is not to be treated as an "indicator" of processes going on at some other level, be it physiological, neurochemical, biophysical (or, especially, mental) even though it is acknowledged that processes are going on at the other physical levels. Just as the biologist knows that quantum mechanical happenings are occurring constantly within and around living things, those happenings generally are ignored. So, too, the behavioral scientist usually ignores physical processes at other levels of investigation. (See comments earlier about constitutive reductionism.)

Another characteristic of the natural sciences is a strong emphasis on interscientist agreement. As noted in the previous section when syntax for theory was discussed, the sciences based in mathematics have a calculus that virtually guarantees agreement. In behavioral science we must rely on language, but in so doing there is no reason not to attempt to employ methods and conventions that are most likely to result in complete agreement. The reason for emphasizing complete interscientist agreement is that methods that promote it are seen to be those that are most useful in leading to effective prediction and control.

The strong emphasis on interscientist agreement is the basis for behavioristic theory's eschewal of intervening variables and hypothetical constructs (MacCorquodale & Meehl, 1948). Intervening variables, unmeasured "variables" that are not assumed to have existence other than in "equations" that relate environmental precursors to behavioral outcomes are viewed generally as unparsimonious, possibly misleading and without logical justification. All these characteristics may lead to disagreement about them. As an example of an intervening variable, consider Tolman's (1932) "expectancy." A rat was said to form an "expectancy" as a result of its experience in a maze, and this expectancy was what allowed the rat to perform efficiently after the requisite experience. Tolman explicitly stated the "expectancy" should not be considered to have physical status, it was merely a useful tool that allowed one to deal with the problem of how the rat could "solve" the maze "problem." Notice that the intervening variable is not parsimonious, it adds nothing to our ability to predict and control and it is not demanded logically. It can be argued, however, that it does serve a heuristic value in that it might lead the experimenter to consider more broadly what the effects of the training history were. That is, by speculating on the nature of the "expectancy" the experimenter might, for example, guess that the training led to a tendency to go toward a certain place in the room, rather than to execute a particular series of turns. The behavioristic objections to intervening variables include a downplaying of the alleged heuristic role. The same experimental questions can be generated without the attendent possible confusions wrought by intervening variables.

Hypothetical constructs, as opposed to intervening variables, are assumed to be potentially observable. These, too, tend to be avoided in behavioristic theory because they are viewed often to be *post hoc* in nature and usually based on everyday preconceptions about behavior. It also can be argued that behavioral science, being in its infancy, is too young to rely heavily on hypothetical constructs.

Despite their criticized status, however, hypothetical constructs do play a role in virtually all behavioristic theories. Even Skinner's theory (1953, 1969, 1974) includes them (e.g., in the form of private stimuli and behavior). The hypothetical constructs deemed allowable in behavioristic theory, however, differ significantly from those espoused by cognitive and other psychological theorists. The hypothetical constructs in behavioristic theories are not given properties that are different from observables and are used mainly in interpretation rather than to guide experimentation. Most importantly, they are viewed as under the control of observable environmental variables. That is, behavioristic hypothetical constructs are not assumed to have autonomous status and therefore are not treated as causes of behavior.

There is, of course, no logical impediment in the use of intervening variables or hypothetical constructs. (Nor is there any logical requirement *for* such entities.) Behavioristic theorists, then, do not make their arguments on the basis of logic, but rather make them on the basis of the historical record. Hypothetical intervening or autonomous causal entities have characterized most of the theorizing about behavior throughout recorded history, yet postulation of such entities has not led to a fruitful science or technology of behavior. In fact, it can be argued (e.g., Skinner, 1953, 1969, 1974, 1977) that postulation of such entities has actually retarded the development of behavioral science. The minimization of the role of hypothetical constructs and intervening variables by behavioristic theorists, therefore, represents a *strategic* choice. (A choice that, incidentally, can be derived from an analysis of scientific verbal behavior [Skinner, 1957].) The behavioristic view is that the understanding of behavior will proceed more rapidly if more attention is paid to manipulable observables and less to "intervening" entities.

The most distinctive characteristic of behavioristic theory is not its insistence on agreement nor its eschewel of hypothetical entities. Rather, its cardinal characteristic is its treatment of causation. In behavioristic theory causes need not be temporally contiguous with effects. That is, behavioristic theory is not tied to "billard-ball causation" (cf. Rachlin, 1974) or what Hume called the "bead theory" of causation. To be comfortable with such a view, it is important first to note that nothing in the definition of "cause" or in its scientific replacement, the functional relation, requires that cause and effect (or independent and dependent variable) be temporally contiguous. It is possible for there to be temporal "gaps" between causes and effects. Most of the causes of behavior in behavioristic theory, in fact, are assumed to act across temporal gaps. This kind of causation has been called "mnemic causation" (Russell, 1921), and can be seen as analogous to the kinds of causes described when physicists speak of "action at a (spatial) distance." To be comfortable with a behavioristic view, then, one must accept the reality of "action at a tempoal distance." Because such a view runs counter to our everyday notions about causation, a behavioristic view on this point is sometimes hard "to sell," yet such an outlook is the very essence of the behavioristic view that important causes of behavior lie in a creature's history. A monkey trained under a fixed-ratio schedule yesterday exhibits characteristic performance today as soon as the experimental circumstances are instituted. Where are the causes of today's performance? For the behaviorist, the important causes include yesterday's training even though there may have been a gap of 24 or more hours between the "cause" and the "effect." For more traditionally oriented students of behavior, it will be presumed that the cause of today's action must precede it immediately and thus we might hear of "expectations" about performance, or "knowledge," or "engrams," or even of "personality variables" as "causes." The behavioristic theorist, as outlined above, sees no advantage, and in fact sees disadvantages, in the postulation of expectancies, knowledge or any other hypothetical entity that bridges the gap between the relevant experience and the subsequent performance. Such entities do not increase our ability to predict and control behavior, and if they are accepted as the primary causes of behavior (in lieu of the critical history) then it becomes less likely that the key aspects of the history will be identified.

The major identifying features of behavioristic theory discussed here—insistence on general interscientist agreement, avoidance of intervening explanatory constructs, and an acceptance of temporal gaps in causal sequences—all can be viewed as rooted in a single viewpoint. The viewpoint is pragmatism (Moore, 1984). The final arbiter for behavioristic theory is the ability to predict and control. On this view, behavioristic "positivism" is a positivism of a very special kind that is justified by an ability to predict and control. A behavioristic theory, therefore, could include, for example, extrasensory perception if that led to better prediction and control. The strategic choices that are inherent in current behavioristic theory reflect the view that, so far, the best prediction and control have arisen from work that emphasizes accurate and precise descriptions and terminology, focuses on directly manipulable variables, and avoids, wherever possible, reliance on unobserved explanatory intermediaries. The argument that is expanded in the next and concluding section of this chapter is that behavioral pharmacology, too, can profit in terms of prediction and control by adopting a behavioristic stance with respect to theory development.

THE NATURE OF A THEORY FOR BEHAVIORAL PHARMACOLOGY

What Kind of Theory Exists Now?

Behavioral pharmacology is not completely without theory. Several "mini-theories" currently play an important role in the science. Three of these are worth special mention. First, the oldest of the theories in behavioral pharmacology is the rate-dependency view. This notion, first proposed by Dews (1958) and then later expanded upon (Kelleher & Morse, 1968; Dews & Wenger, 1977) applies mainly to effects of psychomotor stimulants on free-operant behavior. Across a range of procedures that maintain positively or negatively reinforced free-operant behavior, the effects of a variety of stimulant-type drugs on the frequency of the behavior are predictable on the basis of the baseline (nondrug) frequency of the activity. Despite the fact that rate-dependency can be applied to a more limited range of circumstances and drugs than was originally proposed (cf. Barrett, 1976; McKearney, 1974) and despite the fact that alterative interpretations exist for some of the effects described as rate-dependent (e.g., Branch & Gollub, 1974; Gonzalez & Byrd, 1977), rate-dependency does provide a good description of a substantial body of research (Dews & Wenger, 1977; MacPhail & Gollub, 1975; Sanger & Blackman, 1976). The theory can be criticized as yielding only prediction of a correlation between two dependent variables, but because there are well-established methods for controlling response frequencies (see, for example, Ferster & Skinner, 1957), this theory also points to methods for the control of drug effects. In this vein, it is important to note that the techniques for controlling response rates involve exposing subjects to appropriate *histories*. That is, the explanatory power of the view is behavioral-history dependent.

The two remaining theories to be described have emerged to deal with the phenomenon of drug tolerance. Tolerance refers to the diminished potency of a drug following its (usually repeated) administration. The first of these, the "reinforcement cost" theory, was first put forth by Schuster, Dockens and Woods (1966) and, in its simplest form, states that tolerance to a drug's behavioral effects will develop more fully or more rapidly when the drug's initial effect is to reduce the frequency with which reinforcement occurs. For example, if a subject were responding under a procedure where every 25th response was reinforced (a fixed-ratio, or FR, 25 schedule), and if a particular dose of a drug reduced the response rate (and therefore decreased how frequently reinforcement occurred), the theory predicts that tolerance will develop to the rate reduction. Conversely, if a drug-produced reduction (or increase) in response was not associated with a change in reinforcement frequency (a likely outcome if behavior is maintained by

183

terval schedules of reinforcement, in which availability of reinforcement depends mainly on the passage of time), then, given the absence of other mechanisms for tolerance development, tolerance would not be expected to occur. This theory, then, offers directly means of prediction and control of tolerance-related phenomena. Note that this theory, too, is based on the utilization of behavioral history. A reduction in reinforcement frequency (a key independent variable in the theory) implies a previously "known" level, and this level is the one experienced prior to drug administration (usually during establishment of the behavioral baseline).

The third "mini-theory" is the conditioned-compensatory-response theory of drug tolerance developed by Siegel (1978). This theory is based on the phenomenon of classical (or respondent, or Pavlovian) conditioning. Siegel's theory is that the environment in which drug administration takes place comes to elicit a response (or set of responses) that is opposite to that produced by the drug. Consequently, over the course of repeated drug treatments, the environmentally elicited "counter-responses" block the effect of the drug, with the end result that the drug effect is diminished. The theory also predicts that if the drug is administered in a *new* environment that is sufficiently different from the one in which repeated treatments have occurred, then tolerance will *not* be observed despite the repeated treatments. Several studies have shown that this prediction is born out (Siegel & MacRae, 1984). In this theory, as in the two described previously, behavioral history plays a key explanatory role.

All three of the mini-theories just described have served well as theories. They are testable, relatively simple, are data-derived, and have proven fruitful in generating research examining their generality (and limits). Interestingly, at least from the perspective being promoted in this chapter, is that all three are behavioristic. They rely on objectively measurable parameters as explanations, and they all involve temporal gaps in the causal sequence. The gaps are obvious in the two theories about tolerance. In the reinforcement-cost theory a crucial determinant is the subject's history of exposure to a particular frequency of reinforcement, a history that is not present when the drug exerts its effect. In the compensatory-response theory, it is the history of previous pairings between a distinctive environment and drug administration that is crucial. In the rate-dependency theory, the temporal gap is not so obvious, but it can be argued that here, too, historical factors are paramount, because it is, in the final analysis, these factors that determine nondrug response rate.

The three theories described, despite their limitations, provide excellent guides as to the type of theorizing that is appropriate for behavioral pharmacology. They focus on environmental modification of drug effects and do so without unwarranted (and perhaps unwise) speculation about neuropharmacological "mechanisms." All have been fruitful in the generation of research, and as a group have resulted in integrated bodies of research, so even if they do not withstand the test of time, the data generated as a result of them *and* the theoretical integration they have provided will have to be subsumed by any over-arching theory. That is, these theories, because of their utility in prediction and control, cannot simply be abandoned. They will have to be *incorporated* in or *reduced* to another theory. The argument that is developed more fully here is that this reduction is likely to be most successful if that reduction is of the *homogeneous* type outlined earlier.

Notwithstanding the success of the three mini-theories just discussed, most of the data in behavioral pharmacology do not fall neatly under the umbrella of theory. It may be more accurate to say, metaphorically, that what we currently have is Poincare's "pile of stones." That is, we are still searching for the blueprint to build our house. In several respects then, it may be appropriate to view behavioral pharmacology as "pre-paradigmatic" in Kuhn's (1970) sense. Sciences that are pre-paradigmatic (i.e., those in which a consistent "world-view," or over-arching theory, is yet to be developed), according to Kuhn, are characterized by training of new researchers that is based primarily on the reading of original research rather than textbooks (which hold the "gospel") and by research that is more of the "I am curious about. . . ." nature, than of testing out the ramifications and boundaries of the overall theory. Behavioral pharmacology exemplifies these characteristics.

The Insufficiency of Neuropharmacology

Despite the success of neuropharmacological (usually receptor-based) interpretations of effects in drug-discrimination studies, there is a wealth of data illustrating the inadequacy of neuropharmacological interpretation of behavioral effects of drugs. For example, the oft-demonstrated fact that schedules of reinforcement can drastically modify a drug's behavioral effects (e.g., Dews, 1955; Kelleher & Morse, 1964) presents difficulty for a simplistic receptor-based account. As an illustration, consider the classic demonstration by Kelleher and Morse (1964) that intermediate doses of amphetamine increased the rate of pressing a lever when lever-pressing was maintained by a fixed-interval 10-min schedule of reinforcement but decreased the rate of this same response when it was maintained by a fixed-ratio 30 schedule. To hold to a simplistic receptor-based account would require that the drug interact with one receptor when a fixed-ratio schedule is in effect and with another when a fixed-interval schedule operates. This seems an unlikely possibility.

Accounts based on pharmacological theory also can fall short of being satisfactory even in cases where one might expect them to be appropriate. As an example, it seems reasonable to assume that when combinations of drugs are used, their pharmacological interactions should be the major determinants of the observed outcomes. In fact, in many cases this is true (e.g., Woods et al., 1985). Behavioral factors, however, can be important modifiers of drug-drug interactions. For instance, Rutledge and Kelleher (1965; see Branch, 1974 for a related finding) studied the effects of methamphetamine, pentobarbital and combinations of the two drugs on keypecking by food-deprived pigeons under either a fixed-interval 5-min or fixed-ratio 31 schedule of food presentation. The drugs acted synergistically to increase response rate under the FI schedule yet acted as antagonists under the FR schedule. Thus, the *qualitative* nature of the drug interaction was modified by behavioral variables, an outcome that is not easily explained in simplistic receptor-based terms.

Interpretations based on other pharmacological principles in addition to the concept of the receptor also can be found inadequate when analyzing behavioral effects of drugs. For example, the principles of pharmacokinetics usually are employed to explain the time course of drug action. There is evidence to suggest, however, that the time course of the behavioral effects of drugs cannot always easily be explained by simple (or even complicated) pharmacokinetics. An early hint that this might be the case was provided by Dews (1956) who showed that the time course of recovery of performance following administration of a large dose of phenobarbital to pigeons depended on environmental circumstances. Specifically, he found that performance maintained under a fixed-ratio schedule of reinforcement recovered within 24 hours of drug administration, whereas performance under a fixed-interval schedule took 48 hours to return to normal. These differences appeared despite the absence of any obvious differences in the sensitivity of the two performances to the acute effects of the drug. An even more dramatic finding in this vein was reported by Manning (1973) who studied effects of Δ^9-tetrahydrocannabinol (THC, the major active agent in marijuana) on behavior of rhesus monkeys. Manning's monkeys were trained to press a lever under a procedure in which a food pellet would be delivered if no lever press had occurred for at least 60 s (an interresponse-time-greater-than-60-s, or IRT > 60-s, schedule). Each daily session lasted 3 hours, and in the initial part of the study the drug was administered 3 hours before selected sessions. Manning found that the drug disrupted performance and that it did so unevenly over the 3-hr session. Behavior was considerably more disrupted during the first half of the session than the second half. One interpretation of the change in effect across the session is that it is an illustration of the time-course of action of the drug and is, therefore, governed by the physiological factors involved in absorption, distribution and excretion of the drug. Manning's next experiment, however, revealed that such was not the case. Instead of giving the drug 3 hr before a session, he administered it 4 hr before. The pattern of effects across the 3-hour session was identical to that seen when the drug was given 3 hours before. That is, the change in drug effect across the session depended on exposure to the behavioral procedure and was not simply a result of the passage of time. Obviously, behavioral variables were playing an important role.

The foregoing examples show that for simple drug effects or even effects of drug combinations behavioral factors can play a crucial role. Qualitative as well as quantitative changes in a drug's actions can be effected by behavioral factors, and these changes cannot easily be accounted for by employing pharmacological principles. It is clear, then, that pharmacological theory falls short in providing a complete account of many behavioral effects of drugs. This fact has important implications for the possibility of "reducing" behavioral pharmacology to neuropharmacology (a nonhomogeneous reduction). It was noted earlier that, to be successful, a reduction of one theory to another should exhibit one crucial characteristic—the reducing theory should explain all that was explained by the reduced theory, *and* it should be broader in scope (i.e., it should explain other things, too). By that standard, neuropharmacology should not be considered a candidate for reducing behavioral pharmacological theory because the latter will apply to phenomena that are not explainable by neuropharmacological principles. In a sense, then, the theory to be "reduced," behavioral pharmacological theory, is broader than the reducing theory, neuropharmacology! Of course, a complete description of what happens inside a behaving creature's body as it behaves and as it reacts to drugs, will in some sense eventually provide a "reduction" for behavioral pharmacology, but this will simply be a "constitutive" reduction as described earlier and in no way will render useless or passe a well-developed theory at the level of behavior. In fact, it can be argued that such a behavioral theory is crucial for the success of a constitutive reduction. It will provide the framework for deciding which phenomena are worth describing at the physiological level.

It should be noted here that even research on drug-discrimination, research that heretofore has been explained largely on the basis of receptor pharmacology, is not immune to the influence of behavioral variables. It has been shown, for example, that the conditions of training may result in "biases" towards reporting the presence of the drug when it is not present (McMillan & Wenger, 1984), that stimulus control by the presence of the drug may be overshadowed (cf. Mackintosh, 1974) by the presence or absence of reinforcement (Tomie et al., 1985), and that the breadth of generalization from a training dose to other doses (and perhaps to other drugs?) depends on the magnitude of the training dose (e.g., Kuhn, Appel, & Greenberg, 1974). Such findings indicate that it may be premature, in many cases, to assume that comparable stimulus control exerted by different drugs indicates that a common receptor is involved.

The Place of Pharmacological Theory

Because behavioral pharmacology represents the marriage of pharmacology and experimental psychology (particularly the experimental analysis of behavior), it is clear the pharmacological theory has an important role to play. The purpose of the foregoing descriptions of the limits of pharmacological theory in providing explanations of behavioral effects of drugs was to emphasize that, by itself, pharmacological theory is not enough. Much of pharmacological theory, as it should be, has been derived from idealized preparations in which receptor populations are limited so that clear experiments can be conducted. Experiments in behavioral pharmacology, by contrast, have the potential of being particularly "messy" on the pharmacological side. That is, when a drug is administered to an intact organism and the behavior of the creature is the major focus of attention, it is quite likely that all known types of receptors (and perhaps a few unknown ones) ultimately are involved. This means that pharmacological speculations are risky. Even basically pharmacologically oriented experiments must be interpreted with caution because of potenial "downstream" effects. For example, when comparing two drugs to determine if they exert their actions through the same type of receptor, it may be the case that a drug A binds to receptor X which subsequently activates process P which is mediated by receptor Z. Similarly, drug B may bind to receptor Y and in so doing activates process P. The commonality of effects of drugs A and B then, would not reflect the fact that they bind to the same receptor. Likewise, the fact that effects of both A and B can be blocked by the same drug (a Z blocker) also would not be conclusive evidence that they act on the same receptor. The interpretive problems become even more severe when the effect is "direct" for one drug and "downstream" for the other.

Pharmacologically based interpretations of behavioral effects of drugs, then, are not always adequate and they often entail a considerable amount of risk. Consequently, their role should not be to stand as *the* explanation of effects, but are better viewed as the *starting point* for explanation. For an example of how this might be done, consider again the results reported by Manning (1973) which showed the time course of action of behavioral effects of THC was altered by environmental factors. An important starting point for developing an explanation of the effects would be a description of the pharmacokinetics of THC when administered orally to rhesus monkeys. Such data would provide information on what the time course of action would look like *if behavioral variables played no role*. They would provide an excellent base for describing more precisely the contribution of the behavioral variables. Similarly, drugs that are known to bind to certain types of receptors can be assumed to do so when administered to whole animals (given that it is know that the drug reaches those areas where the receptors exist). Likewise, drugs known to act as antagonists at those receptors also can be assumed to act there. If an antagonism is observed at the behavioral level, a good starting point for an account is in terms of receptor interactions, but to the extent the antagonism depends on environmental factors other explanatory devices will be needed.

It may seem that the foregoing is far from a behavioristic account. Processes as a physiological level are allowed to play an explanatory role. Behavioristic theory, however, as noted earlier, is based primarily on pragmatism. If something allows more accurate prediction and control, then it is not to be avoided simply because it does not fit with someone's preconceptions about what "ought" to be legitimate. The concept of the drug receptor represents an unusual event in science; as noted by Marr (1985) it is "the rare hypothetical construct that made good." It was pointed out earlier that behavioristic theory does not preclude the use of hypothetical constructs. Rather it has very high standards for them, and it appears that the receptor meets those standards.

Goals and Characteristics of a Theory for Behavioral Pharmacology

Now that a role for pharmacological theory has been outlined, the remainder of this section specifies more precisely what the goals of a theory in behavioral pharmacology should be, and what the characteristics of the nonpharmacologic explanatory principles should be like.

One major goal, as emphasized by Carlton (1983), of behavioral pharmacology is the classification of drugs at the behavioral level. Drugs may be classified chemically, but it is quite clear that chemical classification does not provide a very good guide about the possible behavioral effects of drugs. For example, phenothiazines and butyrophenones are quite distinct chemically, yet both are often effective in the treatment of psychotic disorders. Drugs also are classified by their clinical uses, for example, as stimulants and depressants, but these classifications, too, are relatively imprecise. Stimulants sometimes act as depressants and *vice versa*. An alternative to these types of classification that may hold some promise is a classificatory system based on what Thompson and Schuster (1968) called behavioral mechanisms of action. This approach is based heavily on explanatory concepts that have emerged from the experimental analysis of behavior.

There are two major ways that behavioral effects of drugs can be characterized by using concepts from the analysis of behavior. The first is based on the view that a drug may be treated as a stimulus. Stimuli can have a wide variety of behavioral functions. They can act as conditional or unconditional elicitors of behavior, as conditioned or unconditioned reinforcers (either positive or negative), as punishing stimuli or as discriminative stimuli. If a drug is treated as a stimulus, it too may have any or several of these functions in a particular behavioral situation. The levels of complexity involved not only are a reflection of the fact that a drug (as a stimulus) may have several behavioral functions at once, but also of the fact that drugs as stimuli probably are like other environmental events in that they have several aspects, each of which may serve one or more functions in influencing behavior. That is, just as a light source may exhibit intensity, hue, saturation, location, and spectral heterogeneity, a drug as a stimulus too, may have several aspects, any of which is capable of acting as an independent influence. When it can be shown that a drug is serving a particular behavioral function (or set of behavioral functions) an explanation of its effects has been achieved. Recall that explanation involves showing that a particular event is an instance of a more general class of phenomena. Thus, when it is shown that response-dependent delivery of an intravenous dose of a drug serves to increase the subsequent probability of that response, and we say that the drug is acting as a reinforcer, we have provided an explanation of one of the drug's behavioral effects. The power and generality of this explanation, of course, depends on the explanatory strength of the concept of reinforcement. This dependence is discussed in a bit more detail later.

The second way in which drugs can be classified according to behavioral mechanisms of action also involves treating the drug as a stimulus, but in this case the drug is not considered to be taking on or exhibiting a particular behavioral function (although it could be thought of as displaying an effect akin to unconditional elicitation). Instead the drug may be thought of as an internal influence that alters or interacts with ongoing behavioral processes that involve other stimuli, both antecedent and/or consequent. For example, drugs might be classified together on the basis of their ability to diminish the effectiveness of punishment of positively reinforced behavior. Another classification might include drugs that retard the acquisition of conditional reflexes. A careful classification of drugs along these lines could lead potentially to a body of knowledge with enormous practical use if the kinds of behavior for which the drugs are to be used therapeutically can be analyzed into their behavioral constituents. Consider, for example, a futuristic (far fetched?) possibility. Suppose that it was discovered that a certain group of drugs could retard the formation of conditional reflexes that involve noxious unconditional stimuli, i.e., that the drugs lessened the amount of conditioned "fear." Such drugs might be administered to persons who are at risk for the development of phobias.

A behavioral classification of drugs of the type proposed here most assuredly will result in some "overlap." That is, it is quite likely that many (if not most) drugs will fall into several categories. That should be no cause for alarm. Just as the fact that aspirin has antipyretic and antiinflammatory effects in addition to its analgesic ones causes no dismay (instead, it is often viewed as a good aspect) to physicians, so the fact that a behaviorally active drug has a variety of behavioral effects should be no cause for great concern. The important task is to categorize as completely, yet as simply as possible the effects that particular compounds produce.

To categorize drugs in terms of their behavioral mechanisms of action will be far from a simple task for several reasons, yet the potential payoff seems ultimately worth the effort. As Harvey noted years ago (Harvey, 1971), a major problem, perhaps the most significant of problems in pharmacology, is variation in drug response. This is especially true when one speaks of the behavioral effects of drugs. The effect of a drug often varies both within and across subjects. An avenue to identifying a major source of this variability seems one well worth traveling.

The hurdles that stand in the face of the development of a theory in behavioral pharmacology are formidable, and consist of two major impediments. First, the behavioral principles that processes on which the categorization are to be made are in their scientific infancy and consequently are still being developed and refined. It is, therefore, difficult to characterize completely and accurately exactly how a drug interacts with ''basic'' behavioral processes when it is not known precisely what the characteristics of those basic processes are. What will have to be done, then, is something akin to a ''bootstrapping'' operation in which research on drugs not only must concern itself with developing a satisfactory set of classifications, but also must play a role in the development and validation of the *bases* for classification (see Branch, 1984, for additional discussion of the bootstrapping operation). Second, even if behavioral theory were as fully developed as, say, physical theory, the task still would be formidable. Agreement will be needed as to what the critical assay procedures should involve (i.e., what parameters, etc.) and then all the known behaviorally useful drugs would need to be tested. Obviously, all this represents an enormous undertaking, but there is no obvious alternative if we are to understand (and make use of that understanding) drugs that influence behavior.

The type of theorizing about the important behavioral processes, the processes that can provide a rational, useful base for characterizing drug effect on behavior, is an important consideration. The argument here is that such theorizing should follow in the behavioristic tradition. Specifically, such theorizing should focus on observable relationships about which there can be uniform agreement among scientists. In service of this view, it will be necessary to be tolerant of temporal gaps in causal sequences. There *is* agreement among all students of behavior that prior experience plays an important role in the determination of subsequent behavior, so a role for history is well established. At issue is whether conceptual (often mental) entities are useful as bridges across the obvious temporal gaps. The burden of proof lies with those who suggest that such entities are helpful in promoting the development of a science of behavior. The burden is on them for several reasons. One, the addition of hypothetical intermediaries is unparsimonious. Conceptual inventions such as ''expectancies,'' ''knowledge about,'' ''filters,'' ''retrieval mechanisms'' and the like frequently stand only as surrogates for the experiences that led to them. Two, hypothetical intermediaries usually are not very precisely specified. For example, what precisely would ''knowledge about'' a situation entail? Three, such constructions divert attention away from the manipulable causes of behavior. If one is satisfied, for example, that a certain ''expectation,'' usually inferred directly from behavior observed, is the cause of the behavior, one is less likely to examine carefully the experiences that led to ''expectation.'' Four, the success record of hypothetical constructs in furthering our ability to predict and control behavior, is to be charitable, meager. The list of personality constructs, attributional styles, cognitive structures, conceptual nervous activities and the like that have been proposed over the past 100 years as ''explanations'' of behavior is very long. Yet all but the more recent of these inventions have been abandoned. There has been no cumulation or building of a science based on these entities. Instead, one sees a history of total replacement again and again.

In contrast to the unimpressive record compiled by those who champion hypothetical intermediaries, the record of achievement of behavioristic theorizing is enviable. Behavioral principles, though still in their developmental infancy, have been applied with considerable success to improve mental health, education and business to name but a few areas of success. And behavioristic behavioral science has been a cumulative enterprise. The findings and initial generalizations provided by early researchers (e.g., Skinner, 1938) still play an important role in the foundations of the discipline. Current research uses these bases for analyzing and expanding the science to deal with even more complex behavioral phenomena (e.g., Catania, Matthews, & Shimoff, 1982; Hayes, Brownstein, Haas, & Greenway, 1986), and additional refinements of the basic conceptual apparatus continue as well (e.g., Skinner, 1983; Timberlake & Allison, 1974). Behavioristic theorizing, then, has proven its utility and exhibits the characteristics of effective science. Behavioral pharmacology may accelerate the rate of its theoretical development if it adheres to the tenets of behavioristic theorizing.

An often ignored, but perhaps important aspect of theory development in behavior analysis deserves mention. Arguably, one of the most salient features of behavior analytic research and theorizing has been its emphasis on understanding the behavior of *individuals* (cf. Johnston & Pennypacker, 1980; Sidman, 1960). By avoiding the pitfalls associated with being satisfied with effects that occur "on the average" and that are validated *via* tests of statistical significance, behavioristically oriented scientists have been able to rely on the more scientifically (and practically) useful foundation of replication as the key to determining the reliability and generality of behavioral processes. (See Carver, 1978; Gutman, 1977; and Meehl, 1967; 1978 for descriptions of ways significance testing can mislead.) One of the reasons that it has been possible to apply behavioral principles with success is that, by and large, they were discovered and their generality assessed by research that focused on effects in individuals. If theory in behavioral pharmacology is to achieve maximal success, it too should concentrate on effects at the level of individuals.

THE PROSPECTS FOR A THEORY

As noted earlier, behavioral pharmacology currently does not have available a comprehensive theory despite the fact that pharmacological and behavioral theory both have been, and are being, applied regularly with success. There are at least two reasons why this is the case. First, a theory for behavioral pharmacology is going to involve a *blend* of behavioral and pharmacological theory and, as implied by the discussion of the inadequacies of pharmacological theory in dealing with behavioral effects of drugs, this blend is not going to be a simple additive one. The theory will, of necessity, have to be built by delineating the interactions of behavioral and pharmacological processes, and this probably will not be easy. The second, and greater impediment to the development of a comprehensive theory is that behavioral theory is, itself, in need of considerable refinement. The current major concepts in behavioristic theory (e.g., stimulus control, conditioned and unconditioned reinforcement, etc.), although already useful in many circumstances, are too crude to provide a solid base for theory in behavioral pharmacology. Interestingly, some of the inadequacies in behavioral theory have been revealed by research on the behavioral effects of drugs. Any time a drug reveals different effects on two preparations that presumably are illustrations of the same behavioral process, it shows that characterizing the two preparations as the same is an oversimplification (Branch, 1984; Marr, in press). There are many such illustrations (e.g., Barrett, 1976; Branch, Nicholson, & Dworkin, 1977; McKearney, 1974; McKearney & Barrett, 1975).

A theory in behavioral pharmacology, consequently, awaits further development of behavioral theory. Behavioral theory, however, can be advanced by research in behavioral pharmacology; so as mentioned near the beginning of this section, behavioral pharmacology will have to participate in the bootstrapping of behavioral theory. This means that theory development will be promoted if researchers in behavioral pharmacology pay as much attention to the behavioral implications of their work as they do to the pharmacological implications.

Conducting research in the absence of a well-specified theory can be discomforting. The theory that exists currently for behavioral pharmacology might be stated simply as "the environment (broadly conceived to include both past and present ones) can make a difference." It is under this guide that the research must continue. As Poincaré noted, a collection of facts is no more a science than a collection of stones is a house. It is also true, however, that it is not possible to build a house without the "stones." The current role for researchers in behavioral pharmacology is to keep collecting stones with an ever wary eye to finding "keystones" that may allow us to build our house.

REFERENCES

Barrett, J. E. (1976). Effects of alcohol, chlordiazepoxide, cocaine and pentobarbital on responding maintained under fixed-interval schedules of food or shock presentation. *Journal of Pharmacology and Experimental Therapeutics, 196*, 605–615.

Blackman, D. E., & Sanger, D. J. (1978). *Contemporary research in behavioral pharmacology.* New York: Plenum Press.

Branch, M. N. (1974). Behavior as a stimulus: Joint effects of *d*-amphetamine and pentobarbital. *Journal of Pharmacology and Experimental Therapeutics, 189*, 33–41.

Branch, M. N. (1984). Rate dependency, behavioral mechanisms, and behavioral pharmacology. *Journal of the Experimental Analysis of Behavior, 42*, 511–522.

Branch, M. N., & Gollub, L. R. (1974). A detailed analysis of the effects of d-amphetamine on behavior under fixed-interval schedules. *Journal of the Experimental Analysis of Behavior, 21*, 519–539.

Branch, M. N., Nicholson, G., & Dworkin, S. I. (1977). Punishment-specific effects of pentobarbital: Dependency on the type of punisher. *Journal of the Experimental Analysis of Behavior, 28*, 285–293.

Campbell, N. R. (1920). *Physics, the elements.* Cambridge, England: Cambridge University Press.

Carlton, P. L. (1983). *A primer of behavioral pharmacology.* New York: W. H. Freeman.

Carver, R. P. (1978). The case against statistical significance testing. *Harvard Educational Review, 48*, 378–399.

Catania, A. C., Matthews, B. A., & Shimoff, E. (1982). Instructed versus shaped human verbal behavior: Interactions with non-verbal responding. *Journal of the Experimental Analysis of Behavior, 38*, 233–248.

Dews, P. B. (1955). Studies on behavior: I. Differential sensitivity to pentobarbital of pecking performance in pigeons depending on the schedule of reward. *Journal of Pharmacology and Experimental Therapeutics, 113*, 393–401.

Dews, P. B. (1956). Modification by drugs of performance on simple schedules of positive reinforcement. *Annuals of the New York Academy of Sciences, 65*, 268–281.

Dews, P. B. (1958). Studies on behavior: IV. Stimulant actions of methamphetamine. *Journal of Pharmacology and Experimental Therapeutics, 122*, 137–147.

Dews, P. B. (1964). A behavioral effect of amobarbital. *Naunyn-schmiedebergs Archiv für Experimentelleu Pathologie und Pharmakologie, 248*, 296–307.

Dews, P. B., & Morse, W. H. (1961). Behavioral pharmacology. *Annual Review of Pharmacology, 1*, 145–174.

Dews, P. B., & Wenger, G. R. (1977). Rate-dependency of the behavioral effects of amphetamine. In T. Thompson & P. B. Dews (Eds.), *Advances in behavioral pharmacology, Vol. 1*, (pp. 167–227). New York: Academic Press.

Duhem, P. (1954). *The aim and structure of physical theory.* Translated by P. P. Wiener. New Jersey: Princeton University Press.

Efron, D. H. (Ed.). (1968). *Psychopharmacology. A review of progress, 1957–1967.* Washington: U. S. Government Printing Office. USPHS Publication No. 1836.

Ferster, C. B., & Skinner, B. F. (1957). *Schedules of reinforcement.* New York: Appleton-Century-Crofts.

Glick, S. D., & Goldfarb, J. (Eds.). (1976). *Behavioral pharmacology.* St. Louis, MO: C. V. Mosby.

Gonzalez, F. A., & Byrd, L. D. (1977). Mathematics underlying the rate-dependency hypothesis. *Science, 195*, 546–550.

Gutman, L. (1977). What is not what in statistics. *Statistician, 26*, 81–107.

Harvey, J. A. (1971). *Behavioral analysis of drug action.* Glenview, IL: Scott, Foresman.

Hayes, S. C., Brownstein, A. J., Haas, J. R., & Greenway, D..E. (1986). Rules, multiple schedules and extinction: Distinguishing rule-governed from schedule-controlled behavior. *Journal of the Experimental Analysis of Behavior, 46*, 137–147.

Hineline, P. N. (1980). The language of behavior analysis: Its community, its functions, and its limitations. *Behaviorism, 8*, 67–86.

Hineline, P. N. (1984). Can a statement in cognitive terms be a behavior-analytic interpretation? *The Behavior Analyst, 7*, 97–100.

Iversen, S. D., & Iversen, L. L. (1981). *Behavioral pharmacology.* Oxford: Oxford University Press.

Johnston, J. M., & Pennypacker, H. S. (1980). *Strategies and tactics of human behavioral research.* Hillsdale, NJ: Lawrence Erlbaum Associates.

Kelleher, R. T., & Morse, W. H. (1964). Escape behavior and punished behavior. *Federation Proceedings, 23*, 808–817.

Kelleher, R. T., & Morse, W. H. (1968). Determinants of the specificity of behavioral effects of drugs. *Ergebnisse der Physiologie Biologischen Chemie und Experimentellen Pharmakologie, 60,* 1–56.

Kuhn, D. M., Appel, J. B., & Greenberg, I. (1974). An analysis of some discriminative properties of *d*-amphetamine. *Psychopharmacologia, 39,* 57–66.

Kuhn, T. S. (1970). *The structure of scientific revolutions.* Chicago: University of Chicago Press.

MacCorquodale, K., & Meehl, P. E. (1948). On a distinction between hypothetical constructs and intervening variables. *Psychological Review, 55,* 95–107.

Mach, E. (1960). *The science of mechanics.* Homewood, IL: Open Court Press (Originally published in 1885).

MacKintosh, N. J. (1974). *The psychology of animal learning.* London: Academic Press.

MacPhail, R. C., & Gollub, L. R. (1975). Separating the effects of response rate and reinforcement frequency in the rate-dependent effects of amphetamine and scopolamine on the schedule-controlled performances of rats and pigeons. *Journal of Pharmacology and Experimental Therapeutics, 194,* 332–342.

Manning, F. J. (1973). Acute tolerance to the effects of delta-9-tetrahydrocannabinol on spaced responding by monkeys. *Pharmacology, Biochemistry and Behavior, 1,* 665–671.

Marr, M. J. (1985, May). *Behavioral pharmacology: Issues of reductionism and causality.* Invited address at the meeting of the Association for Behavior Analysis, Columbus, Ohio.

Martin, W. R., Eades, C. G., Thompson, J. A., Huppler, R. E., & Gilbert, P. E. (1976). The effects of morphine- and nalorphine-like drugs in the non-dependent and morphine-dependent chronic spinal dog. *Journal of Pharmacology and Experimental Therapeutics, 197,* 517–532.

McAuley, F., & Leslie, J. C. (1986). Molecular analyses of the effects of *d*-amphetamine on fixed-interval schedule performances of rats. *Journal of the Experimental Analysis of Behavior, 45,* 207–219.

McKim, W. A. (1986). *Drugs and behavior. An introduction to behavioral pharmacology.* Englewood Cliffs, NJ: Prentice-Hall.

McKearney, J. W. (1974). Effects of *d*-amphetamine, morphine, and chlorpromazine on responding under fixed-interval schedules of food presentation or electric shock presentation. *Journal of Pharmacology and Experimental Therapeutics, 190,* 141–153.

McKearney, J. W., & Barrett, J. E. (1975). Punished behavior: Increases in responding after *d*-amphetamine. *Psychopharmacology, 41,* 23–26.

McMillan, D. E., & Wenger, G. R. (1984). Bias of phencyclidine discrimination by the schedule of reinforcement. *Journal of the Experimental Analysis of Behavior, 42,* 51–66.

Meehl, P. E. (1967). Theory testing in psychology and physics: A methodological paradox. *Philosophy of Science, 34,* 103–115.

Moore, J. (1984). On behaviorism, knowledge, and causal explanation. *Psychological Record, 34,* 73–97.

Nagel, E. (1949). The meaning of reduction in the natural sciences. In R. C. Stauffer (Ed.), *Science and civilization* (pp. 99–138). Madison: University of Wisconsin Press.

Pickens, R. (1977). Behavioral pharmacology: A brief history. In T. Thompson & P. B. Dews (Eds.), *Advances in behavioral pharmacology, Vol. 1.* (pp. 229–257). New York: Academic Press.

Poincaré, H. (1909). *La science et l'hypothese.* Paris: Ernest Flammarion.

Rachlin, H. (1974). Self-control. *Behaviorism, 2,* 94–106.

Russell, B. (1921). *The analysis of mind.* New York: Humanities Press.

Rutledge, C. O., & Kelleher, R. T. (1965). Interactions between the effects of methamphetamine and pentobarbital on operant behavior in the pigeon. *Psychopharmacologia, 7,* 400–408.

Sanger, D. J., & Blackman, D. E. (1976). Rate-dependent effects of drugs: A review of the literature. *Pharmacology Biochemistry & Behavior, 4,* 73–83.

Schlick, M. (1949). *Philosophy of nature.* Translated by A. von Zeppelin. New York: Philosophical Library.

Schuster, C. R., Dockens, W. S., & Woods, J. H. (1966). Behavioral variables affecting the development of amphetamine tolerance. *Psychopharmacologia, 9,* 170–182.

Seiden, L. S., & Balster, R. L. (Eds.). (1985). *Behavioral pharmacology: The current status.* New York: Alan R. Liss.

Sidman, M. (1960). *Tactics of scientific research.* New York: Basic Books.

Siegel, S. (1978). A pavlovian conditioning analysis of morphine tolerance. In N. A. Krasnegor (Ed.), *Behavioral tolerance: Research and treatment implications* (pp. 27–53). Washington: U. S. Government Printing Office. DHEW publication No. (ADM) 78–551.

Siegel, S., & MacRae, J. (1984). Environmental specificity of tolerance. *Trends in Neurosciences, 7,* 140–143.

Skinner, B. F. (1938). *The behavior of organisms: An experimental analysis.* New York: Appleton-Century-Crofts.

Skinner, B. F. (1953). *Science and human behavior.* New York: Macmillan.

Skinner, B. F. (1957). *Verbal behavior.* New York: Appleton-Century-Crofts.

Skinner, B. F. (1969). *Contingencies of reinforcement: A theoretical analysis.* New York: Appleton-Century-Crofts.

Skinner, B. F. (1974). *About behaviorism.* New York: Knopf.

Skinner, B. F. (1977). Why I am not a cognitive psychologist. *Behaviorism, 5,* 1–10.

Skinner, B. F. (1983). Selection by consequences. *Sciences, 213,* 501–504.

Snyder, S. H. (1984). Drug and neurotransmitter receptors in the brain. *Science, 224,* 22–31.

Stolerman, I. P., & Shine P. J. (1985). Trends in drug discrimination research analyzed with a cross-indexed bibliography, 1982–1983. *Psychopharmacology, 86,* 1–11.

Thompson, T. (1984). Behavioral mechanisms of drug dependence. In T. Thompson, P. B. Dews, & J. E. Barrett, (Eds.) *Advances in behavioral pharmacology, Vol. 4* (pp. 1–45). New York: Academic Press.

Thompson, T., Pickens, R., & Meisch, R. A. (1970). *Readings in behavioral pharmacology.* New York: Appleton-Century-Crofts.

Thompson, T., & Schuster, C. R. (1968). *Behavioral pharmacology.* Englewood Cliffs, NJ: Prentice-Hall.

Timberlake, W., & Allison, J. (1974). Response deprivation: An empirical approach to instrumental performance. *Psychological Review, 81,* 146–164.

Tolman, E. C. (1982). *Purposive behavior in animals and men.* New York: Appleton-Century-Crofts.

Tomie, A., Loukas, E., Stafford, I., Peoples, L., & Wagner, G. C. (1985). Drug discrimination training with a single choice trial per session. *Psychopharmacology, 86,* 217–222.

Turner, M. B. (1965). *Philosophy and the science of behavior.* New York: Appleton-Century-Crofts.

Woods, J. H., France, C. P., Bertalmio, A. J., Gmerek, D. E., & Winger, G. (1985). Behavioral assessment of insurmountable narcotic agonists and antagonists. In L. S. Seiden & R. L. Balster (Eds.), *Behavioral pharmacology: The current status* (pp. 75–92). New York: Alan R. Liss.

Zuriff, G. E. (1985). *Behaviorism: A conceptual reconstruction.* New York: Columbia University Press.

Author Index

A

Abood, L. G., 104, *113*
Abraham, P., *114*
Aghajanian, G. K., 121, *148*, 154, *166*
Agnati, L., 131, *143*, *147*
Ahlenius, S., 82, *113*, 140, *141*, *142*, *148*
Ahmad, A., *114*
Aikawa, J. K., 155, *165*
Alderstein, L. K., 157, 167
Alivisatos, S. G. A., 119, *144*
Allison, J., 192, *196*
Alloway, K. D., 162, *168*
Alvarado-Garcia, R., *118*
Amitai, G., 97, *113*
Annable, L., 154, *165*
Appel, J. B., 16, *37*, 137, 138, *142*, 187, *195*
Aprison, M. H., 83, *114*
Armstrong, J. M., *166*
Arnt, J., 54, 55, *75*, 130, 131, *142*
Arvidsson, L. -E., *142*, *145*
Asarch, K. B., 125, *142*
Asberg, M., 152, *169*
Ashcroft, G. W., 152, *165*
Ashkenazi, A., *116*
Astrachan, D. I., 122, *142*

Attack, C. V., *165*
Awouters, F., *146*
Azmitia, E. C., 119, *142*
Azrin, N. H., 5, *11*

B

Baldesarrini, R. J., 53, *73*, 128, *143*, *148*
Balster, R. L., 6, 12, 86, *114*, 171, 173, *196*
Baker, M., *168*
Barchas, J. D., *168*
Barr, G. A., *166*
Barrett, J. E., 86, 96, 97, 99, 101, *114*, *116*, *118*, 138, *146*, 183, *193*, *195*
Barthelemy, C., 158, *165*, *168*
Baum, W. M., 72, *73*, *76*
Beart, P. M., 156, *166*
Bedard, P., 130, 135, *142*
Bednarczyk, B., 130, 131, *142*, *148*
Beecher, G. D., 65, *73*
Bellenger, J. C., 151, *165*
Belluzzi, J. D., 101, *117*
Bendotti, C., 140, *142*, *147*
Bensch, K. G., 161, *165*
Bernard, C., 1, 2, 5, 6, 8, *11*

Berlyne, D. S., 59, *73*
Berryman, R., 23, *37*
Bertalmio, A. J., *196*
Bertilsson, L., 152, *169*
Bevan, P., 45, *74*
Biel, J. H., 104, *113*
Bignami, G., 82, 95, 97, 98, 101, *114*
Binnis, J. K., *165*
Birdsall, N. J. M., 80, *114, 115*
Birdsall, T. G., 39, *76*
Blackman, D. E., 171, *193, 195*
Blasberg, R., 150, *165*
Blau, A. D., *166*
Block, M. C., 40, *73*
Bloom, F. E., 10, 12, 40, 59, *74*
Boadle-Biber, M. C., 155, *165*
Bockaert, J., *168*
Borbely, A. A., 153, *165*
Boren, J. J., 96, 97, *114*
Boren, M. C. P., 20, *37*
Borsini, F., 147
Boyar, W. C., *146*
Boyd, E. S., 83, 85, *117*
Bradley, P. B., 120, *142*
Bradshaw, C. M., 45, 58, 61, 65, 66, 72, *73, 74, 76*
Brait, K. A., 160, *166*
Branch, M. N., 3, 5, *12*, 171, 183, 185, 191, *193, 194*
Bridger, W. H., *166*
Brown, G. L., 151, *165*
Brown, J., 130, *142, 144*
Brownstein, A. J., 192, *194*
Bruce, A., 152, *167*
Bruckstein, R., *113*
Bruckwich, E. A., *168*
Brunswick, D. J., 126, *148*
Buckley, N. J., 80, 106, *114*
Bunney, W. E., *165, 168*
Burgen, A. S. V., 80, *115*
Burleigh, D. E., 85, *114*
Burnstock, G., 80, 106, *114*
Butcher, L. L., 81, *118*
Byrd, L. D., 62, *75*, 173, 183, *194*

C

Caan, A. W., *166*
Cabbat, F. S., 161, *166*
Callahan, P.M., 137, *142*

Callaway, E., 158, *168*
Campbell, N. R., 174, *194*
Capon, D. J., *116*
Carbera, R., 83, *114*
Carlsson, A., *142, 143, 145*, 150, *165*
Carlton, P. L., 81, 82, 95, 98, *114*, 172, 183, *194*
Carney, J. M., 99, *116*
Caron, M. G., 155, *168*
Carroll, F. I., 108, *114*
Carter, D. A., 41, *74*
Carver, R. P., 192, *194*
Cassella, J. V., 140, *143*
Catania, A. C., 192, *194*
Caufield, M. P., 80, 107, 108, *114*
Centore, J. M., 161, *168*
Cervo, L., 128, 140, *142*
Chait, L. D., 86, *114*
Chalmers, R. K., 85, *114*
Chiang, P. K., 95, *114, 118*
Cho, A. K., 92, *114*
Chouinard, G., 154, *165*
Chutkow, J. G., 155, *165*
Clark, A. J., 52, *74*
Cleland, G., 45, *74*
Clemens, J. A., *143*
Clody, D. E., 53, *75*
Collins, K. R., 41, *75*
Colmenares, J. L., 150, *166*
Colpaert, F. C., 130, 138, *142, 146, 148*
Conn, P. J., 120, 121, 128, *142*
Conner, J. E., 122, 124, 130, *143, 147, 148*
Conrad, D. G., 45, *74*
Conway, P. G., 126, *143, 148*
Cook, D. G., 160, *166*
Cook, L., 100, *115*
Cooper, A. J., 152, *166*
Cooper, J. R., 10, 12, 59, *74*
Coppen, A., 152, 154, *166*
Cornes, S. J., 130, *142*
Cortes, R., 80, 111, *114*, 121, *147*
Cote, M., 156, *169*
Coulter, J. D., 151, *166*
Cox, B. M., 161, *168*
Crawford, T. B., *165*
Creese, I., 59, *74*, 155, 156, *166, 169*
Crisp, T., 163, *169*
Cumming, W. W., 23, *37*
Cunningham, K. A., 137, 138, *142*
Curzon, G., 122, 128, 140, *143, 145*, 150, *166*

D

Dackis, C. A., 158, *166*
Dale, H. H., 79, *115*
Damiano, B. P., 124, *147*
Dashwood, M. R., 122, *143*
Datta, S. R., 152, *166*
Davey, G., 45, *74*
Davis, A. J., 57, *74*
Davis, B. M., *115*
Davis, J. L., 131, *145*
Davis, J. N., *165*
Davis, M., 122, 123, 140, *142, 143,* 151
Davidson, A. B., 100, *115*
Deakin, J. F. W., 122, *143*
De Angelo, T. M., 124, *146*
De Feudis, F. V., 82, *115*
De Souza, R. J., 127, 135, *144*
deWit, H., 40, *76*
Dews, P. B., 1, 4, *12,* 13–16, 21, 24, 32, 34, 35, *37,* 62, *74,* 149, *166,* 172, 173, 183, 185, 186, *194*
de Villiers, P. A., 45, 57, 67, *74*
De Vries, D. J., 156, *166*
Dickinson, S. L., 122, *143*
Dockens, W. S., 183, *196*
Domino, E. F., 80, 82, 83, 85, 92, 102, *115, 116, 117*
Donahoe, T. P., 128, *145*
Dourish, C. T., 140, *145*
Drens, A. T., 92, *116*
Drust, E. G., 122, 124, 130, *147,* 148
Duhem, P., 176, *194*
Dunlap, C. E., 161, *168*
Dutta, S. N., 82, *116*
Dworkin, S. I., 5, *12,* 193, *194*
Dykstra, L. A., 7, 12, 16, 37, 81, 82, 95, 104, *117, 118*

E

Eades, C. G., *195*
Eberle, K. M., 130, *145*
Ebert, M. H., *165*
Eccleston, D., *165*
Eckstein, F., 81, *118*
Edelman, A. M., *168*
Efron, D. H., 171, *194*
Egozi, Y., 83, *116*
Eichelman, B., 151, 152, *167*

Eison, A. S., 137, 140, *143*
Eison, M. S., 137, 140, *143*
El Mestikawy, S., 120, *144*
Emerit, M. B., 120, *144*
Engel, G., 120, 126, 128, *142*
Engel, J. A., 140, *143, 145*
Enjalbert, A., *168*
Enwonwu, C. O., 161, *166*
Erickson, C. K., 85, *114*
Ernouf, D., *165*
Ervin, F. R., 151, *168*
Essman, W. B., 155, *166*
Ettenburg, A., 40, *74*
Evans, H. L., 32, 38, 65, *74*

F

Fahn, S., 160, *166*
Fallon, S. L., *146*
Farrell, J. P., 154, *166*
Feniuk, W., *142*
Fernandez-Gvasti, 140, *141*
Fernstrom, J. K., 150, *166*
Ferraris, A., *147*
Ferster, C., 1, 3, *12,* 19, *37,* 183, *194*
Fibiger, H. C., 40, 41, 66, 67, *74,* 77
Filewich, R. J., 59, *74*
Finnerty, R. J., 137, *144*
Fischman, M. W., 40, *74,* 137, *147*
Fisher, A. G., 40, *73*
Fisher, L. A., 151, *168*
Foders, R. M., 79, *116*
Forler, C., 122, *148*
Fowler, S. G., 41, 43, 59, *74, 75*
Fozard, J. R., 120, 121, 122, 137, 141, *142, 143, 146, 148*
France, C. P., *196*
Franklin, K. B. J., 57, 58, *74*
Fraser, C. M., 106, *115*
Frazer, A., 120, 121, 123–125, 128, 131– 133, 135, 136, *143, 145–147*
Fremming, K. H., 154, *168*
Friedman, S., 161, *167*
Fuller, R., 140, *143*
Fuxe, K., 131, *143, 146*

G

Gabay, S., 119, *144*
Gaddum, J. H., 119, *143*

Galbicka, G., 96, 98, 104, 106
Gallager, D. W., 154, *166*
Gallistel, C. R., 40, 57, 58, *74, 75*
Galzigna, L., 161, *166*
Garcia-Valdez, K., 157, *167*
Gardiner, T. W., 161, *166*
Gardner, C. R., 129, *144*
Gardner, M. L., 80, *117*
Garreau, B., 158, *165, 168*
Garritini, S., *147*
Gelperin, A., 119, *145*
Gendelman, D. S., 140, *143*
Gendelman, P. M., 140, *143*
Genovese, R. F., 16, *37*
George, S. R., 156, *169*
Gerber, G. J., 40, *76*
Gerhardt, S., 67, *75, 76*
Gerson, S. C., 128, *143*
Gessa, G., 151, *169*
Giachetti, A., 80, 107, *115, 116*
Gibbons, J. L., 150, 151, 152, *166*
Gilbert, P. E., *195*
Gillin, J. C., 128, *144*
Gilman, A. G., 35, *38*
Glennon, R. A., 120, 137, 138, 139, *143,
    144, 146, 148*
Glaeser, B. S., *146*
Glick, S. D., 172, *194*
Glossmann, H., 155, *166*
Glusman, M., *166*
Gmerek, D. E., *196*
Gold, M. S., 158, *166*
Goldberg, H. L., 137, *144*
Goldberg, M. E., 83, *115*
Goldberg, S. R., 80, *117*
Goldfarb, J., 172, *194*
Gollub, L. R., 20, *37*, 173, 183, *194, 195*
Gonzalez, F. A., 62, *75*, 173, 183, *194*
Goodwin, F. K., 151, *165, 168*
Goodwin, G. M., 127, 135, *144*
Gordon, R. K., 95, *118*
Gorzalka, B. B., 140, *146*
Gothert, M., 120, *143*
Goyal, R. K., 80, *115*
Goyer, P. F., 151, *165*
Gozlan, H., 120, *144*, 146
Gramling, S. E., 41–43, *74, 75*
Grahame-Smith, D. G., 122, 128, *144*, 151,
    152, *166*
Green, A. R., 122, 124, 127, 129, 135, *143,
    144*

Green, D. M., 16, *37*
Green, R. A., 128, *144*
Greenberg, I., 187, *195*
Greengard, P., 155, 167
Greenwald, B. S., *115*
Greenwald, D., 151, *167*
Greenway, D. E., 192, *194*
Grier, J. B., 19, *37*
Griffith, R. C., *114*
Griffiths, W. J., 151, *166*
Gudelsky, G. A., 127, *144*
Gustafson, J. A., 131, *143, 147*
Gutman, L., 192, *194*
Guy, A. P., 129, *144*

H

Haas, J. R., 192, *194*
Haber, B., 119, *144*
Hacksell, V., *142, 145*
Hall, D. P. Jr., *115*
Hall, J. E., 124, *144*
Hall, M. D., 120, *144*
Hamblin, M. W., 156, *166*
Hamilton, A., 53, 54, 56, 58, *75*
Hamon, M., 120, *144, 146, 168*
Hammer, R., 80. 107, 108, *115*
Handley, S. L., 130, 131, *142, 144, 145*
Haroutunan, Y., *115*
Hart, E. B., *75*
Hartman, E., 151, *167*
Harvey, J. A., 128, *146, 147*, 190, *194*
Haslett, W. L., 92, *114*
Hauck, A. E., 138, *143*
Hayes, S. C., 192, *194*
Heal, D. J., 127, 131, *143, 145*
Hegstrand, L. R., 151, 152, 155, *167*
Heikkila, R. E., 161, 163, 164, *167*
Heise, G. A., 16, *37*, 81, 82, *115*
Heller, A., 81, 82, 113, *117*
Hemrick-Luecke, S. K., *143*
Henderson, L. J., 163, *169*
Henzel, W., *116*
Herbet, A., *168*
Herrera-Marschitz, M., 53, *75*
Herrington, R. N., 152, *167*
Herrnstein, R. J., 1, 39, 44, 45, 57, 72, *74,
    75*
Herz, A., 95, *115*
Herz, J. M., *113*

Herzberg, B., 152, *166*
Heuring, R. E., 120, *145*
Heyman, G., 40–45, 50–53, 56, 58, 66, 70, 75
Higgins, G. A., 107, *114*
Hilbert, R. P., 152, *169*
Hilderbrand, R. L., 152, *169*
Hillenbrand, K., 120, *143*
Hineline, P. N., 179, *194*
Hirota, T., 59, *73, 75*
Hirsch, M. J., 150, *166*
Hjorth, S., 123, 128, 140, *141–143, 145*
Hoffstetter, A., 95, *115*
Hole, K., 151, *167*
Holm, A. C., *147*
Holz, W. C., 5, *11*
Holzman, S., 6, *12*
Hornung, R., 155, *166*
Horvath, E., 80, *117*
Horvath, T. B., *115*
Horwitt, M. K., 162, 167
Hoyer, D., 120, *143, 145, 147*
Huey, L., *115*
Hull, J. H., 45, *75*
Hulme, E. C., 80, *114, 115*
Humphrey, P. P. A., *142*
Huppler, R. E., *195*
Huston, P. H., 128, *145*
Hyttel, J., 54, 55, *75*, 130, *142*

I

Issodorides, M. R., 119, *144*
Iversen, L. L., 59, 75, 80, 82, 107, 111, *115*, 172, *194*
Iversen, S. D., 59, *75, 172, 194*
Izenwasser, S. I., 157, *167*

J

Jackson, A., 122, *143*
Jackson, D. S., 65, *73*
Jacobs, B. L., 119, 122, 125, *145, 148*
Jacoby, J. H., 150, *166*
James, W., 39, *75*
Janssen, P. A. J., 130, 138, *142, 146*
Janowsky, D. S., 83, 92, *115*
Jarvik, M. E., 23, *37*
Jenden, D. J., 92, *114, 116*

Jenney, E. H., 83, 92, *116*
Jimmerson, D. C., *165*
Johanson, C. E., 137, *147*
Johns, C. A., 80, 82, *115*
Johnson, H. E., 83, *115*
Johnston, E. C., 152, *167*
Johnston, J. M., 192, *194*
Jolly, D., 66, *75*
Jonsson, G., 131, *143, 147*
Jorgensen, A., 52, 53, *76, 77*
Joseph, M. H., 150, *166*

K

Kakiuchi, S., 155, *167*
Kalkman, H. O., 120, *145*
Kandel, E. R., 113, *115*
Kanoff, P. D., *115*, 155, *167*
Kantak, K. M., 150–153, 156–160, *167*
Karlen, B., 89, *115*
Karras, D., 40, 57, 58, *75*
Kass, E., 122, *142*
Katz, J. L., 16, 19–31, 37, 81, 99, *114, 118*
Kaufman, S., 150, 161, *167*
Kawada, S., 161, *168*
Kehne, J. H., 140, *143*
Kehr, W., *165*
Kellar, K. J., 81, *115*
Kelleher, R. T., 1, 21, 38, 62, 76, 81, 99, *115, 173, 183, 185, 194, 195*
Kennedy, B., *115*
Kennett, G. A., 140, *145*
Kerlavage, A. R., 106, *115*
Kidd, E. J., 137, *148*
Kinzie, D. L., 40, *75*
Kirk, L., 53, *76*, 154, *168*
Klein, W. J., *165*
Klemfuss, H., 122, *145*
Knaak, J. B., 83, *115*
Knapp, S., 151, *169*
Knott, P. J., 150, *166*
Koenig, I. D. V., 59, *73*
Koenig, J. I., 127, *144*
Koerner, O., 161, *165*
Komlos, M., 161, *169*
Koob, G. G., 40, *74*
Koss, F. W., 107, 108, *115*
Kotin, J., *168*
Krnjevic, K., 80, *115*
Kruesi, M. J. P., 149, *167*

Kuhn, D. M., 187, *195*
Kuhn, T. S., 185, *195*
Kurz, H., 95, *115*

L

Lader, M. H., 152, *167*
Laduron, P. M., 120, *145*
Lajtha, A., 150, *165*
Lal, H., 82, *117*
Lambrecht, G., 85, 107, *117, 118*
Landfield, P. W., 156, 157, *167*
Langley, J. N., 79, *115*
Larsen, J. J., 130, *142*
Larsson, K., 82, *113,* 140, *141, 142*
Laties, V. G., 15, 21, 32, 35, *38*
Leach, K., 106
Leander, J. D., 6, 12, 82, 95, 99–101, 104, *116, 118*
Leberer, M. R., 59, *74*
Lebovitz, R. M., 130, *147*
Lebrecht, V., 135, *145, 148*
Leccese, A. P., 154, *167, 169*
Leddet, I., *165*
Lefkowitz, R. J., 155, *168, 169*
LeLord, G., 158, *165, 168*
Leslie, F. M., 161, *168*
Leslie, J. C., 173, *195*
Lester, B. K., 151, *166*
Leysen, J. E., 120, *145, 146*
Liao, R. M., 43, *74*
Lieberman, H. R., 149, *168*
Liebman, J. M., 67, *75, 76*
Liebowitz, S. F., *166*
Liljequist, S., *143*
Lindberg, P., *142, 145*
Lindquist, M., *165*
Liretto, A., 156, *169*
Logan, F. A., 45, *76*
Lohman, W., 161, *165*
Lorens, S. A., 128, *145*
Loukas, E., *196*
Lovenberg, W., *168*
Lucki, I., 65, *76,* 121, 123–131, 133, 135–139, *143, 145–147*
Luz-Chapman, S., *113*
Lyness, W. H., 154, *167, 168, 169*
Lyon, M., 59, 61, *76*
Lyon, R. A., 120, *148*
Lytle, L. D., 151, *168*

M

Maayani, S., 83, *116*
MacCorquodale, K., 180, *195*
MacDougal, E. J., *165*
Mach, E., 10, *12,* 175, *195*
MacKintosh, N. J., 187, *195*
MacPhail, R. C., 183, *195*
MacRae, J., 184, *196*
Maggs, R., 152, *166*
Maina, L., 161, *166*
Maj, J., 131, *146*
Makk, G., *168*
Mandell, A. J., 151, *169*
Manning, F. J., 186, 188, *195*
Mansbach, R. S., 138, *146*
Manzino, L., 161, *167*
Marcinkiewicz, M., 121, *146*
Markowitz, R. A., 86, 96, 101, 102, *116, 118*
Marr, M. J., 2, *12,* 189, 193, *195*
Marsden, C. A., 151, *167*
Martin, L. L., *146*
Martin, W. R., 173, *195*
Martineau, J., 158, *168*
Martino, A. M., *115*
Mason, N. R., *143*
Matthews, B. A., 192, *194*
Matthews, W. D., 130, 131, *146*
McAuley, F., 173, *195*
McDowell, J. J., 72, *76*
McKearney, J. W., 33, 38, 104, *116,* 183, 193, *195*
McKenney, J. D., 138, *144, 146*
McKim, W. A., 98, *116,* 172, *195*
McKinney, M., 107, *116*
McMaster, S. B., 99, *116*
McMenamy, R., 150, *168*
McMillan, D. E., 82, 98, 99, 100, 101, *116,* 187, *195*
McSweeney, F. K., 44, 70, *76*
Meehl, P. E., 180, 192, *195*
Meert, T. F., 138, *142*
Meisch, R. A., 171, *196*
Meltzer, H. Y., 127, *144*
Mendelson, S. D., 140, *146*
Mennini, T., *147*
Mercer, E. H., 10, *12*
Messing, R. B., 151, *168*
Metha, P., 80, *115*
Michatek, H., 82, 95, 98, 101, *114*
Micheletti, R., 107, *116*

Miczek, K. A., 98, 101, *116*
Middaugh, L. D., 163, *169*
Middlemiss, D. N., 120, 129, 137, *142, 146,*
    148
Milar, K. S., 16, *37*
Miller, H., *168*
Miller, N. E., 36, *38*
Milner, G., 162, *168*
Minugh-Purvis, N., 130, 135, *145, 146*
Modigh, K., 128, *146*
Moerschbaecher, J. M., 33, *38*
Mohs, R. C., *115*
Moller, S. E., 154, *168*
Monaghan, M. M., 41–45, 50, 53, 70, *75*
Montagna, E., 107, *116*
Moore, J., 182, *195*
Morand, C., 151, *168*
Morgan, G. A., 156, 157, *167*
Morley, H. J., 58, *76*
Morrison, J., 80, *117*
Morse, W. H., 1, 15, *37,* 62, *76,* 81, 99,
    100, *115,* 173, 183, 185, *194, 195*
Moser, V., 85, 107, *117, 118*
Muh, J. P., 158, *165, 168*
Mullikin, D., 155, *168, 169*
Murphy, D. L., 152, *168*
Muscat, R., 40, *76*
Mutschler, E., 85, 107, *117, 118*
Mylecharane, E. J., *142*

N

Nagel, E., 2, *12,* 177, 178, *195*
Nahorski, S. R., 120, 126, *146*
Nakashima, Y., 161, *168*
Navarro, A. P., 95, *114*
Neale, R. F., 120, *146*
Neill, J., 129, 137, *148*
Nelson, D. L., 120, 124, *146, 147,* 155, *168*
Neuhaus, H. U., 153, *165*
Nevin, J. A., 23, *37*
Nicholson, G., 5, *12,* 193, *194*
Niemegeers, C. J. E., 120, 130, 138, *142,*
    145, 146
Nilsson, J. L. G., *142, 145*
Nilvebrant, L., 106, *116*
Nobler, M. S., 121, *146*
Norman, D. A., 18, *38*
Nowack, J. Z., 135, *145*

O

Offord, S. J., 120, 125, 128, 131, *143, 146,*
    147
Ogren, S. -O., 130, 131, *143, 147*
Oksenberg, D., 126, *147*
Olds, M. E., 82, 83, 85, 102, *115, 116*
Oncly, J., 150, *168*
Ordway, G. A., 120, *147*
Osborne, N. N., 119, *147*
O'Shaughnessy, K. M., 131, *147*
Overton, D. A., 137, *147*

P

Padilla, F., *114*
Palacios, J. M., 80, 111, *114,* 120, 121, *147*
Palider, W., 131, *146*
Pare, C. M., 154, *168*
Parent, M., 55, *76*
Parham, K., *114*
Pasternak, G. W., 155, *168*
Pauling, L., 162, *168*
Pazos, A., 120, 121, *147*
Pears, E., 45, *74*
Pedigo, N. W., 120, 125, *147*
Pennypacker, H. S., 192, *194*
Peoples, L., *196*
Peralta, E. G., 106, 111, *116*
Perez, L. A., *118*
Perez-Cruet, J., 151, *169*
Peroutka, S. J., 120, 125, 126, 130, 131, 135,
    145, 147, 148
Pert, A., 160, *168*
Pert, C. B., *168*
Peterson, G. L., *116*
Peterson, R. E., 150, *169*
Pfeiffer, C. C., 83, 92, *116*
Phebus, L., 151, *168*
Phillips, A. G., 41, 66, 67, *74*
Philpot, J., 131, *145*
Picarelli, Z. P., 119, *143*
Pichat, L., 120, *144, 146*
Pickens, R., 62, *76,* 171, *195, 196*
Pickering, R. W., 130, *142*
Pierson, M. E., 138, *144*
Pilc, A., 135, *148*
Pinchasi, I., 83, *116*
Pitt, B., 162, *168*
Poincaré, H., 174, *195*

Pollitt, N., 162, *168*
Potegal, M., *166*
Pradhan, S. N., 82, *116*
Presek, P., 155, *166*
Prowse, J., 67, *75*
Pycock, C. J., 130, 135, *142*

R

Rachlin, H. A., 72, 73, *76*, 181, *195*
Raese, J. D., 155, *168*
Ramachandran, J., *116*
Ransom, R. W., 125, *142*
Rattan, S., 80, *115*
Rawlow, A., 131, *146*
Rebec, G. V., 162, 163, *166, 168*
Rees, A. R., 124, *144*
Rees, D. C., 15, *38*
Reichenberg, K., 130, *148*
Riblet, L. A., 137, *143*
Richard, M. M., *114*
Richardson, B. P., *142*
Richelson, E., 107, *116*
Ringdaghl, B., 92, *116*
Risch, S. C., *115*
Robbins, T. W., 59, 62, *76*
Rokosz, A., 130, *148*
Rosenblatt, J. E., *168*
Rosecrans, J. A., 83, 85, 92, *116*, 138, *144*
Ross, E. M., 35, *38*
Ross, S., *166*
Roth, R. H., 10, *12*, 59, *74*
Rouot, B. M., 155, *169*
Ruddle, H. V., 45, 61, *73, 74*
Rumney, L., 161, *166*
Russell, B., 182, *195*
Russell, R. W., 81, 82, 98, 113, *116*
Rutledge, C. O., 21, *38*, 185, *195*

S

Salvaterra, P. M., 79, *116*
Samada, H., 161, *168*
Saminin, R., 128, 140, *142, 147*
Sanchez, D., *142, 145*
Sanders-Bush, E., 120, 121, 128, *142*
Sanger, D. J., 171, *193, 195*
Saxena, P. R., *142*
Schaefer, A., 161, *169*

Scatchard, G., 52, *76*
Schechter, L. E., 140, *147*
Schimerlik, M. I., *116*
Schlick, M., 175, *195*
Schlicker, E., 120, *143*
Schlosberg, A. J., 128, *147*
Schuster, C. R., 35, *38,* 40, *74,* 137, *147,* 172, 183, 189, *196*
Schwartz, R. D., *115*
Seeman, P., 156, *169*
Seiden, L. S., 6, *12,* 40, 66, *75,* 81, 82, 95, *117,* 171, 173, *196*
Seoane, J. R., 156, *169*
Seregi, A., 161, *169*
Setler, P. E., 40, *77*
Shaw, D. M., 152, 154, *166*
Sheard, M. H., 151, *169*
Shepard, G. M., 10, *12*
Shih, J. C., 125, *142*
Shimoff, E., 192, *194*
Shine, P. J., 173, *196*
Shizgal, P., 57, *75*
Sidman, M., 2, *12,* 45, *74,* 192, *196*
Siegal, S., 184, *196*
Sills, M. A., 120, 124, 125, 128, 129, 133, *146, 147*
Simansky, K. J., 140, *147*
Simmons, K., 149, *169*
Singh, A. N., 55, 56, *76*
Singh, L., 130, 131, *144, 145*
Sinton, C. M., *146*
Sivit, C., *168*
Sjoqvist, F., 89, *115*
Sjostrand, L., 152, *169*
Skinner, B. F., 1, 3, 8–10, *12,* 19, 35, *37, 38, 76,* 181, 183, 192, *194, 196*
Slangen, J. L., 111, *117, 118*
Sloviter, R. S., 122, 124, *147, 148*
Smith, C. B., 21, *38*
Smith, C. D., 130, 131, *146*
Smith, D. G., *169*
Smith, D. H., *116*
Smith, F. L., 154, *169*
Smith, L. M., 125, *147*
Snoddy, H. D., *143*
Snowman, A. M., 155, *168*
Snyder, S. H., 120, 130, 135, *147,* 155, *168, 169,* 173, *196*
Snyderman, M., 45, *76*
Sokolovsky, M., 83, *116*
Sokomba, E., 162, 163, 164, *169*

Sourkes, T. L., 154, *165*
Spealman, R. D., 80, *117*
Spector, R., 161, *169*
Spencer, D. G. Jr., 82, 107, *117*, 138, *148*
Spindler, J., 40, *76*
Spinweber, C. L., 152, *169*
Sprouse, J. S., 121, *148*
Stafford, I., *196*
Stanky, M., 137, *143*
Stanton, J. B., *165*
Stark, P., 83, 85, *117*
Stauning, J. A., 53, *76*
Stellar, J. R., *75*
Stein, J. M., 150, *167*
Stein, L., 101, *117*
Stewart, R. M., 128, *148*
Stitzer, M., 80, *117*
Stolerman, I. P., 173, *196*
Stone, G. A., *146*
Stone, G. C., 99, *117*
Straughn, D., 80, 107, *114*
Subramanion, N., 161, *169*
Suzve, R., 161, *168*
Svensson, L., 140, *142, 143, 148*
Swets, J. A., 16, *37, 39, 76*
Szabadi, E., 45, 58, 61, 66, 72, *73, 74, 76*

T

Tagliamonte, A., 151, *169*
Tagliamonte, P., 151, *169*
Tanner, W. P., Jr., 39, *76*
Taylor, P., 80, 81, 85, *117*
Taylor, R. L., *115*
Terpstra, G. K., 111, *117, 118*
Teschemacher, H., 95, *115*
Teshima, Y., 155, *167*
Thomas, T. N., 163, *169*
Thompson, D. M., 33, *38*
Thompson, J. A., *196*
Thompson, R. F., 113, *117*
Thompson, T., 1, 3, *12,* 16, *35,* 171, 172, 173, 178, 189, *196*
Timberlake, W., 192, *196*
Tischler, M. D., 140, *143*
Titeler, M., 120, 125, *144, 148*
Titus, E., 150, *169*
Tobler, I., 153, *165*
Tolbert, L. C., 163, *169*
Tolman, E. C., 180, *196*

Tomie, A., 187, *196*
Tondo, L., 126, *148*
Torrance, R. W., 83, *114*
Toussaint, C., 55, *76*
Towell, A., 40, *76*
Traber, J., 80, *117,* 138, *148*
Traskman, K., 152, *169*
Traskman, L., 89, *115*
Tricklebank, M. D., 122, 123, 126, 129, 137, 138, *148*
Trulson, M. E., 122, *148,* 163, *169*
Turner, M. B., 175, 176, *196*
Tyce, G. M., 155, *165*

U

Udenfriend, S., 150, *169*
Ungerstedt, U., 53, *75*
U'Pritchard, D. C., 155, *169*
Ursin, R., 152, *169*
Usdin, T. B., 155, 156, 160, *169*

V

Vaillant, G. E., 83, 92, *117*
Van Neuten, J. M., 120, *145*
Venter, J. C., 106, *115*
Verge, D., *146*
Vetulani, J., 130, 131, 135, *142, 148*
Vilter, R. W., 161, *169*
Viveros, H., 83, *114*

W

Wagner, G. C., *196*
Walters, J. K., 151, *169*
Wambebe, C., 162, 163, 164, *169*
Wang, H. L., 125, *146*
Warbritton, J. D. III, 128, *148*
Ward, H. R., 124, *146*
Warner, B. T., 130, *142*
Wasley, J. W. F., *146*
Watanabe, M., 156, *169*
Wayner, M. J., 150, *167*
Wedeking, P. W., 100, *117*
Weinberger, S. B., 151, *169*
Weiner, N., 80, 81, 104, *117*
Weiss, B., 15, 21, 35, *38,* 81, 82, 113, *117*

Weissbach, H., 150, *169*
Wenger, G. R., 16, *37*, 62, *74*, 83, 85, *117*, 183, 187, *194, 195*
Wess, J., 85, 107, 111, *117, 118*
Whitman, J., 151, *167*
White, L. K., 162, *168*
Wieland, S., 127, 130
Wightman, R. M., *166*
Wiles, D., 52, 77
Wilkinson, G. N., 46, *76*
Willcocks, A. L., 120, 126, *146*
Williams, L. T., 155, *169*
Williams, M., *146*
Willner, P., 40, 66, *76*
Wilkstrom, H., *142, 145*
Winger, G., *196*
Wise, R. A., 40, 76, 101, *117*, 154
Wistedt, B., 52, 77
Witkin, J. M., 33, *38*, 81, 83–88, 90–111, *114, 116, 118*
Witkin, K. M., *118*
Witter, A., 111, *118*
Wolfe, B. B., 120, *147*
Woolf, N. J., 81, *118*
Wood, R. W., 15, *38*

Woods, J. H., 6, *12*, 183, 185, *196*
Wren, W. H., 140, *143*
Wurtman, R. J., 150, *166*
Wyatt, R. J., 128, *144*

Y

Yamamura, H. I., 120, *147*
Yamazaki, R., 155, 167
Yeomans, J. S., 57, *75*
Young, R., 138, *144*
Young, S. N., 151, 154, *165, 168, 169*
Yu, D. S. L., *169*

Z

Zarevics, P., 40, 77
Zeigler, M., *115*
Zeiler, M., 3, *12*
Zemp, J. W., 163, *169*
Zis, A. P., 40, 77
Zuriff, G. E., 179, *196*

Subject Index

A

Acetylcholine, 79
Acquisition, 81
Adiphenine, 95–99, 105
AF-DX 116, 111
Aggression,
  modulation by magnesium, 156, 157
Alpha-flupentixol, 40
Alprenolol, 125, 126
Alzheimers, 80, 82, 111, 112
Amphetamine,
  interactions with magnesium, 159
  matching law, 58–62, 68, 69, 72
  schedule-controlled responding, 185
  serotonin syndrome, 122
  stimulus control, 22, 23, 25, 27–32
Analgesia, 7, 8
Anticholinesterase, 80, 83
Antidepressants,
  anticholinergic activity, 81
  chronic administration, 133–138
  depression, 154
  matching law, 66, 67
  serotonin, 119, 128, 131
Antipsychotic, 40
Anxiety, 15, 119, 139
Anxiolytic,
  punished responding, 5, 100, 101
  serotonin, 128

Apomorphine, 156
Aprophen, 95–101, 105
Arecoline, 80, 95
Ascorbic acid,
  behavioral effects, 162
  interactions, 163
  neurochemistry, 161, 162
Atropine,
  interaction with physostigmine, 102, 103
  muscarinic antagonist, 80
  role in oxotremorine toxicity, 92, 93
  schedule-controlled responding, 99, 100,
    102–105
Attention deficit disorder, 165
Avoidance,
  effects of chlorpromazine, 15
  interactions with magnesium, 156
  matching law, 67–72
  muscarinic drugs, 83–92, 98, 107
Azaprophen, 95–100, 105, 107, 108

B

Behavioral history, 4, 8, 9, 13, 35
Behavioral mechanisms, 4, 5, 9, 23, 34–36,
    72, 81, 172, 189, 190
Benactyzine, 80, 93–97, 104, 105
Benzodiazepines,
  drug discrimination, 138

207

Benztropine, 93, 94
Bethanechol, 80, 84
Bias, 19
Brain stimulation,
   amphetamine, 72
   antidepressants, 66, 67
   behavioral pharmacology, 81
   matching law, 44, 56, 57
   muscarinic drugs, 104
   neuroleptics, 57
   reinforcement, 40
Buproprion, 66, 67
Buspirone,
   anxiety, 125, 140
   drug discrimination, 137–139
   serotonin syndrome, 124, 125

C

p-chloramphetamine, 122
Chlordiazepoxide, 101
m-Chlorophenylpiperazine (m-CPP), 120, 124,
   128, 133
   drug discrimination, 138
Chlorpromazine,
   matching law, 46, 48–59, 69, 70, 72
   role in behavioral pharmacology, 172
   stimulus control, 13–15
Cholinesterase, 80, 83
Cis-flupentixol, 46, 53, 59, 73
Clock stimuli, 15
Clonidine, 130
Cocaine,
   aggression, 159
   chronic administration, 158, 159
   stimulus control, 22, 23, 25, 27
   with magnesium, 158, 159
Conditional discrimination, 21, 23, 25, 28, 33,
   34
Conjunctive schedule, 25, 34
Context, 4
Contingencies of reinforcement, 9
Cyproheptadine, 154

D

Depression,
   in matching law, 66, 72
   role of tryptophan, 151, 155

Deprivation, 41, 45, 57, 71
Desipramine, 66, 67, 131, 133
Dexetimide, 106
Diazepam, 69, 70
Diet,
   behavioral effects, 149–164
5,7-Dihydroxytryptamine, (5,7-DHT), 131,
   132, 135
   aggressive behavior, 151
Diisopropylphosphofloridate, 80
2,5-Dimethoxy-4-bromoamphetamine (DOB),
   124, 136, 138
2,5-Dimethoxy-4-iodoamphetamine (DOI),
   124, 138
2,5-Dimethoxy-4-methylamphetamine (DOM),
   124, 138
Discrete trial, 16
Discriminative control, 13
Dopamine, 53–56, 59, 61
   and serotonin syndrome, 122
Drug discrimination, 6
   role in behavioral pharmacology, 173
   serotonin, 137, 140

E

Electroconvulsive shock, 135, 151
Ethylaprophen, 95
Experimental analysis of behavior, 1, 2, 5, 8,
   171
Extinction, 40, 41, 98

F

Fenfluramine, 122
Fixed interval,
   muscarinic drugs, 96, 101
   neuropharmacology, 105
   stimulus control, 13, 15, 17, 19–28, 30–32
Fixed ratio, 13, 99, 154
Fluoxetine, 131
Fluphenazine, 46, 52, 54
Formalistic fallacy, 35

G

Gepirone, 137, 138, 140

Printed and bound by CPI Group (UK) Ltd, Croydon, CR0 4YY

17/10/2024

01775685-0003

H

Hallucinogens, 124
Haloperidol, 159
History,
  behavioral, 4, 8, 9, 35, 39
  drug, 4, 8, 9
5-Hydroxytryptamine (5-HT), 119–141
  autoreceptors, 126
  behavioral syndrome, 122–126
  diet, 150–152
  drug discrimination, 137–140
  feeding, 119, 139, 151
  head shaking, 130–131
  sexual behavior, 139, 140, 151
  sleep, 151
  startle, 139, 140
  temperature regulation, 126–128
  tryptophan, 150
  unconditioned behaviors, 121–131
5-Hydroxytryptamine 1A (5-HT$_{1A}$),
  anxiety, 128
  locomotor behavior, 128–131
  receptor subtype, 120
  syndrome, 123–126, 132
  temperature, 126–128
5-Hydroxytryptamine 1B (5-HT$_{1B}$), 133–135
  locomotor activity, 135
5-Hydroxytryptamine 1C (5-HT$_{1C}$), 129,
  135
5-Hydroxytryptamine 2 (5-HT$_2$),
  depression, 133–136
  feeding, 140
  head shaking, 130–131
5-Hydroxytryptamine 3 (5-HT$_3$), 139
8-Hydroxy-2-(di-n-propylamino) tetralin (8-
  OH-DPAT),
  depression, 133
  receptor ligand, 120
  serotonin syndrome, 123–126
  temperature regulation, 127, 128, 135
  tolerance, 133

I

Ipsapirone,
  anxiety, 125, 127, 140
  drug discrimination, 137–139

K

Ketanserin,
  drug discrimination, 138
  5-HT$_2$, 120, 121, 125, 129, 130

L

Levetimide, 106
d-Lysergic acid diethylamide (LSD), 123, 124,
  141

M

Magnesium,
  behavioral effects, 156
  dopamine binding, 155
  interactions with drugs, 158–160
  serotonin binding, 155
Matching law, 39, 41–73
Matching-to-sample, 23
McN-A-343, 109, 111
Mecamylamine, 95
Mechanism of action,
  behavioral, 4, 5, 9, 23, 34–36, 72, 81
Memory, 81, 111, 159
Meperidine, 104
Mesulergine, 120
Metergoline, 121, 125, 128
Methacoline, 85
Methiothepin, 127
5-Methoxy-N,N-dimethyltryptamine (5-
  MeODMT), 124, 127, 128, 130, 133
Methylatropine, 83, 86, 89 91, 95, 96, 107,
  111
Methysergide, 121, 125, 154
Mianserin, 120, 128, 129, 131
Morphine, 104
Motor performance,
  matching law, 40, 41, 43–45, 50, 52, 58,
    59, 61, 62
Muscarinic, 79–113
Multiple schedule, 20, 29, 33, 56, 100

N

Naloxone, 104
Neostigmine, 83, 89

Neuroleptics, 40, 46–58, 72
Neurotoxicity, 92–95
Nicotine, 103
Nicotinic, 79–113
Nomifensine, 66–68

O

Opiate, 6, 7
Oxotremorine, 80, 84, 86–95, 99, 101, 102, 104, 109–112
Oxotremorine-M, 85, 88, 89, 109–112

P

Parkinsonian, 59, 81
Pentobarbital, 1, 21–32, 100, 173
Phenothiazine, 53, 189
Physostigmine, 80, 83–92, 102–104
Pigeons, 17, 44
Pilocarpine, 80, 95
Pimozide, 46–51, 55, 72, 129
Pindolol, 120, 121, 125–128
Pipamperone, 121, 125
Pirenperone, 130
Pirenzepine, 95, 105, 107–111
Prazosin, 129
Promazine, 21–23, 25–27, 32
Propranolol, 120, 125–128
Psychophysics, 16
Punishment, 5, 81, 100, 101, 139
Pyridostigmine, 85

Q

Quipazine, 124

R

Rate dependency, 3, 16, 62–66, 173, 183
Receptor, 6, 10, 52, 59, 79
Reductionism, 3, 5, 11, 177
Reinforcement,
  contingencies, 9
  efficacy, 41, 42, 44, 46, 52, 53, 55, 63, 72
  frequency, 8
  processes, 40, 58, 73
  rate of, 3, 41, 43, 46, 49, 59, 65, 69, 71

Reinforcer,
  type, 57, 82
Response,
  duration, 85, 86
  effort, 40
  rate, 4, 13, 33, 43, 45, 59, 62, 67, 71
Ritanserin, 120, 138
RU 24969, 120, 124, 129, 138, 139, 140
  drug discrimination, 137, 138

S

Scatchard plot, 51
Schedules of reinforcement, 3, 4, 82, 185
Schizophrenia, 55, 155
Scopolamine, 80, 93, 94, 98, 104
Self-administration,
  tryptophan and d-amphetamine, 154
  5,7-DHT, 154
Sexual behavior, 139, 140
Signal detection, 39
Spiperone, 120, 125, 126
Squirrel monkeys, 68, 83–92, 96–105, 111, 112
Startle, 139, 140
Steady state behavior, 8
Stimulus control, 3, 15–36

T

Tardive dyskinesia, 160
Temperature regulation, 126–128, 139
$\triangle^9$-Tetrahydrocannabinol (THC), 187
Tolerance, 183, 185
Tranylcypromine, 135
Trazodone, 131
Tolerance,
  to serotonin agonists, 133, 134
1-(m-Trifluoromethylphenyl)piperazine (TFMPP), 120, 124, 128, 133
  drug discrimination, 138
Tryptophan,
  aggression, 151
  feeding, 151
  sexual behavior, 151
  sleep, 153

V

Variable interval, 41, 58, 65–68